Table of Contents

The Sleep Book for Tired Parents

Written by Rebecca Huntley

Illustrations by Kathleen Kerr

SOUVENIR PRESS

Acknowledgements

This book is dedicated to my own children who inspired finding new solutions, to all the families who shared their experiences, and to those families who are looking forward to more restful sleep.

I gratefully acknowledge the patient editing of Shari Steelsmith, the technical support of Carol Bysinger and Amby Schultz, and the honest feedback from readers who offered insights at various stages.

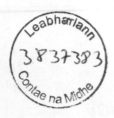

Copyright © 1991 by Parenting Press, Inc.

The right of Rebecca Huntley to be identified as author of this work has been asserted by her in accordance with the Copyright, Designs and Patents Act 1988.

First published in the USA by
Parenting Press, Inc., Seattle

First British Edition published 1992 by
Souvenir Press Ltd.,
43 Great Russell Street, London WC1B 3PA
This edition, completely reset, published 1997.
Reprinted 2004

ISBN 0 285 63703 7

Typeset by Galleon Typesetting, Ipswich
Printed in Great Britain by
Creative Print & Design Group (Wales), Ebbw Vale

INTRODUCTION

The basic premise of this book is that sleep problems are as unique as the individuals involved. There are no blanket answers. Instead, there are choices. The most successful solution is the one that:

- fits the problem
- fits the people involved
- people are committed to.

Too often parents try too many things and pile up a list of failures, or are immobilized because they feel they won't be able to 'tough it out'. Decisions and actions come more easily when your alternatives and goals are clear.

This book is designed to give you that information and take you through the problem-solving process.

First, you will gain a solid base of information about children's sleep – and the problems that can develop. You will look at typical problems and begin to identify issues that concern you. There are suggestions and tips to try. You will look at ways other families have gone through the problem-solving process. Four major approaches, as devised by child development experts, are outlined so you can begin to assess what might work best for your family.

The discussion focuses not only on the child but also on the parent. It recognizes that parents struggle both with the problem and with implementing the solution. It will help you explore your feelings and reach a state of readiness to work on the problem.

Then, you are encouraged to develop an individualized plan – tailored to your specific problem, family values and lifestyle, and long-range goals. Sleeping well doesn't always 'just happen'. It is a skill that can be learned and can be taught in the way you, as a parent, find most comfortable.

How to use this book. This book moves from the general

to the specific. The exercises will help you apply the information to your own situation and begin the problem-solving process. Some exercises you will 'think through'. Others need a written response. The information builds upon itself. Since this is a complex issue, some topics will be covered in more than one place. An effort has been made to direct you to the related sections.

Some problems can be addressed with relatively simple interventions. Others take a well thought-out plan. The four major approaches are outlined in the Summary Sheets in the appendices. They are for quick referral while carrying out your plan. It is recommended that you read the entire book before beginning to make changes.

Chapter 1 SLEEPLESS NIGHTS

Children's sleep, or the lack of it, is a major preoccupation for many of today's parents. 'Does your child sleep through the night yet?' seems to be the first question everyone asks – if your puffy eyes do not speak for themselves. Someone else's smug response, 'My child has slept through the night ever since we brought him home from the hospital,' wakes up every hair on the back of your neck – even though they, like the rest of your body, can barely function.

It is, understandably, an issue charged with an entire range of emotions – anger, guilt, relief, and elation. All parenting issues seem intensely important, but this one seems even more so. Perhaps this is because sleep – or the need for it in both parent and child – can begin to affect one's decision-making ability and undermine even the most confident parent. It can bring discord to ordinarily happy families and affect parents' feelings towards their child.

But it is possible to look objectively at the problem, to define it as it appears in your family, and to determine a course of action with which you will feel comfortable. In order to devise a workable plan, you first need some solid information about young children's sleep.

What is a Sleep Problem?

When a child's sleep habits cause recurring or continuing problems for the child or his parents, there is a sleep problem.

Types of Sleep Problems

Sleep problems vary in cause, duration, and ages they affect. Still, they fall into categories with typical characteristics and have variations on the basic themes. Some children have only one type of problem. Others demonstrate several types at the same time. For still others, the type of problem might be related to the child's development and will change as he

7

grows and faces new experiences. Knowing where your child fits will help you describe the specific behaviours that are causing problems and give you clues as to how to respond.

Frequent Waking

Elizabeth is nine months old and I haven't had a full night's sleep since she was born.

Frequent waking is a problem when a child wakes more than you expect for her developmental level – or more than you can tolerate. This may be once or several times a night.

She might never have developed the pattern of sleeping for a long stretch or never learned to get back to sleep after normal night-time arousals. The problem might be related to difficulty getting to sleep alone. She may have learned to need and expect help from her parents to get back to sleep. Or new night waking might be stimulated by illness, dreaming, or developmental disequilibrium. In those cases, she may need to re-learn getting herself back to sleep for a long stretch.

Waking for Feeding

I give him a bottle and he goes right back to sleep, but I wonder if he really needs it.

Some infants simply sleep through the expected feeding time, others continue waking long after what seems developmentally appropriate. This child never learns the pattern of sleeping a long stretch. He requires food to satisfy 'learned hunger' or requires sucking and comforting to get back to sleep.

Difficulty Getting to Sleep

After the third glass of water, I'm ready to scream!
She is afraid of the monsters in her cupboard.

This problem can affect all ages. Bedtime is drawn out and battles get worse and worse. Parents cajole, threaten, and bribe, and then they wonder how things got so out of control. There can be many reasons for this, including fears, separation anxiety, and simply not having learned the skill of getting to sleep on one's own.

Difficulty Sleeping Alone

To avoid a big chase, we just lie down with him until he falls asleep.

There are degrees of parental involvement in the bedtime process. It becomes a problem when it takes too much time or the parent begins to feel burdened or manipulated. It also becomes a problem when a parent's involvement, or lack of involvement (for whatever reason), keeps the child from getting to, or back to, sleep. This can be an unexpected culprit in frequent waking – when he needs something from his parent in order to go back to sleep.

Unusual Sleep Cycles

She is just not ready to go to sleep – but we are!

Sleep patterns follow an internal set of rhythms. When they are skewed early, or late, or are extremely irregular, it becomes a problem because the child does not mesh with the family routine. Very often a problem at one end of the day begins to affect the other end or the remainder of the day. When a child's apparent sleep needs (much more, or much less) are different from her parents', it can also cause a problem.

Nightmares and Sleep Terrors

He wakes up screaming and really seems terrified.

Nightmares and sleep terrors are often confused because the incidents can look so similar. The child 'wakes' with confusion and fear once or several times a night. However, there are definite differences between a nightmare and a sleep terror. Recognizing them is crucial because the best response is very different for each.

Does Your Child Have a Sleep Problem? Refer to the definition of sleep problem: *When a child's sleep habits cause recurring or continuing problems for him or for his family, then there is a sleep problem.*

The best way to identify a possible problem is to listen to the parents – yourselves. Listen to how *you* describe the

---

EXERCISE 1.1: Types of Problems

The following checklist will help clarify the type or types of problem your child is having. Mark each sentence that generally describes your child. Use a check mark for those that fit at some times. Circle that check mark if it is a current issue.

_____ 1. She wakes during the night and can't find her dummy.

_____ 2. The only way I can get him back to sleep is to feed him.

_____ 3. He sleeps in late and won't take a nap.

_____ 4. She hops out of bed defiantly.

_____ 5. He wants several drinks of water and goodnight kisses.

_____ 6. She comes to our bed during the night.

_____ 7. I can't wake him in the morning.

_____ 8. He won't be alone in his room because of the 'monsters and snakes'.

_____ 9. She comes to our room scared and crying.

_____ 10. He needs to have all the lights on at bedtime but will look at books forever if I let him.

_____ 11. She screams and thrashes around.

_____ 12. My husband can't put her to bed – she only wants Mum.

_____ 13. We are ready for bed, but he is not!

_____ 14. He calls out during the night wanting juice.

_____ 15. She wakes up several times with no particular pattern.

_____ 16. He seems to wake about every few hours.

_____ 17. He is reluctant to go to sleep at bedtime because he's afraid of bad dreams.

Note any uncircled check marks; these indicate changes – possibly improvements. Fit your answers into the following key to see possible types of problems your child shows. There may be come overlap because the same symptom can be an indicator of several types of problems.

Frequent waker: 1, 6, 9, 14, 15, 16
Night feeder: 2, 14
Unusual sleep cycle: 3, 7, 10, 13, 15
Nightmares and sleep terrors: 8, 9, 11, 17
Difficulty getting to sleep: 4, 5, 8, 10, 12, 13, 17
Difficulty sleeping alone: 4, 5, 6, 8, 9, 12, 15, 16

experience of parenting. How quickly, or how often, does the subject of sleep come up? How much energy do you spend thinking, worrying, or complaining about sleep? Are your feelings about your child being coloured by your frustration and exhaustion? If there were just one thing you could change about your child or your life, would it be sleep?

The fact that there is a problem may seem obvious to you; or, you may find yourself wavering. Perhaps you blame yourself, or maybe after a 'good night' you think it's really not so bad. Exercise 1.2 may help you clarify your thinking or make up your mind.

Your own description is better than any clinical definition. As you read this book you will continue to describe your situation. Problem areas and choices for solutions will become more clear.

Why Work On It?

The bags under your eyes, the weight you have been losing or gaining, the grumpiness and sheer exhaustion – these are the obvious reasons to make some changes. Your child's physical and emotional well-being are also reasons.

Dr Burton White, author of *The First Three Years of Life*, feels that sleep problems understandably occur in families where children are loved and whose needs have been met. So, in some ways, the emergence of sleep problems is not necessarily a bad sign. He notes that it is the *continuance* of sleep disturbances that can cause deeper problems.[1]

Dr Marc Weissbluth, author of *Healthy Sleep Habits, Happy Child*, states that the development of healthy sleep habits is *not* automatic. If your child has not learned them, then his functioning during wakefulness is not 'optimal'.[2] Put simply, a sleep-deprived child (waking several times a night or missing out on even an hour) is not at his best. His cognitive processes will be fuzzy and his social functioning will be marked by grumpy unpredictability.

A child can 'adjust' to whatever sleep patterns he has fallen into. (Look at how *you* have 'adjusted'. Do you say 'I didn't know it was possible to exist with so little sleep'?) However, there are signs – some subtle, some blatant – that he is not at his best.

EXERCISE 1.2: Does My Child Have A Sleep Problem?

If you are wondering if your child's sleep habits qualify as a 'problem', you might want to consider the following issues. Mark each statement **A** (agree) or **D** (disagree). If yours is a two-partner family, it is helpful if both partners mark the statements separately to see how each of you feels about the situation.

_____ 1. I feel my child is not getting enough sleep. He is irritable during the day and shows subtle signs of lack of sleep.

_____ 2. My child wakes too early or goes to sleep too late.

_____ 3. Sleep seems frightening to my child.

_____ 4. My child wakes during the middle of the night.

_____ 5. I wonder if my child is eating too much or too frequently.

_____ 6. Bedtime is unpleasant for my child. She goes to bed angry, sad, over-stimulated, or frightened.

_____ 7. I believe an undesirable pattern may be developing.

_____ 8. My child needs me at times that seem unreasonable to me. I fear he may be overly dependent on me.

_____ 9. Bedtime is unpleasant. I dread it.

_____ 10. I usually feel deprived of sleep. I crave a night of undisturbed sleep.

_____ 11. I need to go to bed sooner than I would like in order to accommodate an early riser or a non-sleeper.

_____ 12. My fatigue or anger is affecting my relationship with my child, his siblings, or my partner.

_____ 13. The current situation feels out of control.

_____ 14. I find myself asking, 'Is my child the only one acting like this?'

_____ 15. My child continually disturbs the rest of the family.

Some of these statements reflect the child's behaviour. Others reflect the family's response. If you agreed with three or more, there is definitely a problem within the family system. This checklist is only a guideline. A child may show only _one_ area of difficulty that turns the family upside down. Go back to the definition of a sleep problem. If you experience it as a problem, then it is a problem worth working on.

It is the parents' job to insist on healthy sleep, just as they insist on healthy nutrition, to give the child the strongest base from which to grow.

Good sleep habits do not necessarily happen spontaneously. This is a skill that can be learned by children and facilitated by parents.

Children are individuals. Each one brings to the issue of sleep his own needs, personality, and physical functioning. This does not mean that you need to accept your child's sleep patterns as 'the way it is'. Your goal as parents is to help your child fit smoothly into your family – and into his world. You can recognize his uniqueness, while teaching him skills to make his life easier.

Commonly, after the sleep issue is resolved, parents notice real differences. The child is more easy-going, less frustrated, happier, and more predictable. Parents wonder why they didn't do something sooner. Parents, too, feel more content and self-confident.

In the long run, the child's sense of independence and self-esteem is enhanced. When he masters sleep problems, he has mastered an important part of life. (He knows it is important by the significance you – and the rest of the world – have placed on it.) Sleep and night-time can be frightening; children need to know that Mum and Dad are in charge.

A child who continually disrupts his parents' sleep forms an unhealthy view of life. He learns that his needs are the *only* important ones. This is a far cry from what parents intend.

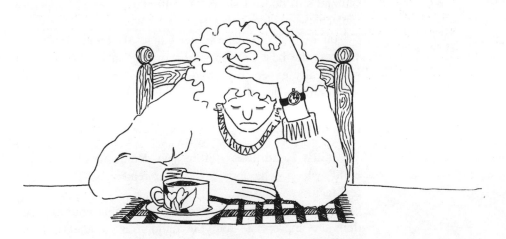

"Who, me? Sleep deprived?"

Perhaps this is the message you would like to send:

*I love you and I want you to grow up to be a
happy person. Sleeping is part of life. The way
you are sleeping now doesn't fit with the rest of
our family. It is becoming a problem for us all.
Let's work on it together.*

In Practical Terms:

Reasons to make some changes:

- Your family life does not run smoothly because of disrupted sleep.
- You are exhausted and frustrated with yourself and your child.
- You feel out of control.
- You suspect your child's moods are being affected by lack of sleep.
- You want him to be at his best when he is awake.
- You feel your child is forming an unnatural view of life. You are concerned that she is developing life-long habits that may be debilitating or unhealthy.

When is the Right Time?

Friends are saying, 'That child is running your life.' Others are saying, 'She will start sleeping better soon – just be patient.' Then you hear the dreaded, 'My child is three years old and still doesn't sleep.' You think, that *can't* happen to me! That *won't* happen to me!

You are ready to make some changes. But you wonder . . . when is the best time to start working on it? When can I realistically expect my child to make some changes? The answer to the question 'when' is a complex one and must be examined on two levels: a child's readiness and the parents' readiness.

Child's Readiness. Before you decide to change your child's sleep behaviour review her readiness. There are a few factors to consider.

Check developmental stage. Be certain that your expectations are appropriate for your child's developmental level. Know what is considered 'average' for your child's age. For example, when you learn that most two year olds need a nap, you will feel more confident in expecting one. Although you can take preliminary, stage-setting steps beforehand, a child might not have the neurological maturity to sleep all night until he is six months old. Do not feel burdened by norms, but use them as guideposts.

TABLE 1.1: Developmental Expectations

Problem:	Developmental Issues:
Frequent Waking	An infant may need to be six months old before gaining the neurological maturity necessary to settle into an 8–10 hour night-time stretch of sleep (although many do it sooner). Older children tend to wake periodically due to illness, dreams, or while learning a new developmental task. Very often the cause is undetermined.
Waking for Feeding	After three or four months, a healthy, full-term infant no longer needs night feedings for nutritional reasons. Early risers may wake up hungry.
Difficulty Sleeping Alone	Separation issues peak at times of developmental disequilibrium (leaps or regression). Typical times: four to six months, nine to twelve months, one and a half to two years, and subsequent half-year stages. Fears are strong for toddlers and preschoolers. Older preschoolers tend to fall asleep quickly once settled.
Unusual Cycles	An Infant may have his 'days and nights mixed up' – this can be adjusted. Up to and including nine months, an infant may take a third nap around dinner time, so a late bedtime is not inappropriate. Typical bedtime for a toddler/preschooler is between 7:30 and 9:00 p.m.
Nightmares	Infants appear to 'dream' (or to be affected by dreaming) at around 9 months. Children continue to gain the language to express dreams and fears beginning at age two. This may peak during preschool years.
Sleep Terrors	These are probably experienced by infants, occur most commonly around age four, and decrease by school age.

Consider temperament. Personality or temperament should also be taken into consideration – especially during developmental upheaval, when getting through a typical day is a feat. Generally, this would not be a logical time to introduce new expectations.

Other factors. Never begin a new programme when a child is ill or is dealing with other changes – for example, a new house or a new sibling. Try to consider the whole situation, but if there never seems to be a 'right' time, you may be making too many allowances. There will never be the perfect time; you may just have to plunge in. Children are incredibly resilient and adaptable.

**Parents'
Readiness**

This 'Readiness Factor' has more to do with the success of all of the methods than any other factor. This cannot be emphasized enough and should certainly not be scoffed at.

Too often parents will succumb to feelings of guilt or to pressure from other people. They try something – usually whatever has been 'suggested' most often – and it fails. The list under 'we-tried-that' only looks like proof that nothing will ever work.

All methods of addressing sleep problems are difficult even when begun with the utmost determination. To begin before you are ready is to set yourself – and your child – up for failure. That sense of failure usually lasts longer than if you had waited until you were fully ready.

How do you know when you are 'ready'? It is a balance of being exhausted, frustrated, and prepared.

Developing a plan that feels personalized to your situation will give you more confidence to begin. Deciding what does and doesn't feel right about the current situation helps you define the problem for yourself. Trouble-shooting for 'glitches' before you encounter them gives you more ammunition. *Working with your partner ahead of time* builds a stronger, united front. Finding supports before you need them means they will be there when you do. Examining the range of emotions and thoughts you have on the whole issue will help you give yourself permission to begin. You need to reach the conclusion that it is important to make some changes.

Is it Too   *At five months I thought she was too young to sleep better. At*
Late?   *seven months she was learning to crawl – and was <u>so</u>*
                frustrated. At a year she wouldn't leave my side. Now she's
                two and teething miserably again. Before I know it she'll be
                in college – I guess then it's okay to stay up all night!

Is it too late? 'She climbs out of her crib,' 'He can cry for hours,' 'She still nurses every two hours,' 'He has a baby brother now,' the reasons to take, or not to take action are many.

It is never too late – you only have more information to take into account. Maybe it would have been easier yesterday, but chances are it will be easier today than tomorrow.

Summary   Identifying problem areas and your motivation for making changes are the first steps in problem solving. You also need solid information about children's sleep. This will be discussed in the next chapter.

Chapter 2 BUILDING THE BASICS

Most of the information parents have on the subject of sleep is second hand – someone else's success or horror story. The information, most often, is conflicting and produces feelings of guilt.

My mum says she gave all of us kids cereal at about four weeks and never had any trouble with our sleeping.

There is a body of knowledge that you will find helpful. This chapter will discuss some of what is known about children's sleep.

Sleeping Through the Night

'Sleeping through the night' is a phrase that is probably best banned from our vocabulary. Let's face it, *no one* really sleeps through the night. If you poll a group of adult friends and ask them how they slept last night, you will undoubtedly hear such things as:

The wind woke me up.

At 3:00 a.m. I looked at the clock and was relieved to see I had two more hours before the alarm would ring.

If you poll a group of parents, and get past the 'She has always slept through the night,' you will hear a variety of comments:

When he is teething, he has a little trouble sleeping.

She seems so hungry at around 2:00 a.m. – must be a growth spurt.

He has been waking with bad dreams.

If sleeping all night long, every night, is your expectation for your child, you may be setting yourself up for frustration. Sleep needs and patterns change with age,

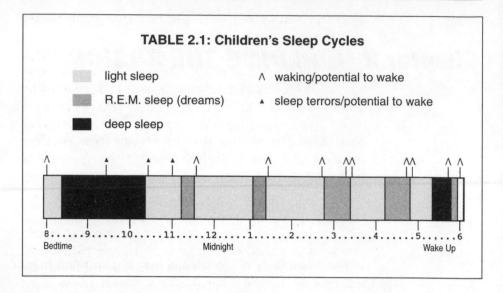

TABLE 2.1: Children's Sleep Cycles

illness, and emotional or even environmental factors. Just as with other parenting issues, our goals, expectations, and approaches must be constantly re-evaluated.

It is misleading to think of sleep as a state we simply fall into at night and wake from in the morning. Sleep research has shown that there are definite patterns and fluctuations during the night. They play important roles to help refresh us and can reveal some causes behind sleep disturbances.

The descriptions of these cycles can be quite technical. Because a basic understanding is crucial, an effort has been made to give a very simple explanation of what occurs and how your child might be affected.

All people – children and adults – move through distinctly different sleep states which progress from drowsiness to very deep sleep. In the *waking state* we are rational and functional. In *non-REM sleep* the body rests and restores itself. In *REM sleep* the mind is active again and dreaming occurs. (*REM* stands for 'rapid eye movement' – a stage of sleep that is characterized by such eye movement.)

The night begins as the child moves quickly through drowsiness and into deep sleep within ten minutes. Waking a child in deep sleep might be almost impossible – this is the time your child can be moved from the car or your arms into bed without waking.

Deep sleep makes up the next two or so hours of sleep. After about an hour (and again after the next hour), it is interrupted by a brief arousal when the child seems to be sleeping and waking at the same time. Behaviours range from crying out or opening eyes to the more extreme thrashing about. *It is during this arousal that confused thrashing, sleep terrors, sleep walking, or bedwetting might occur.* Although we tend to think that these behaviours are a result of dreaming, that is not the case since dreaming does not occur until *REM sleep*.

The bulk of the remaining night is spent moving between light sleep and the *REM* episodes in which dreaming occurs. There is a tendency to wake briefly while changing states – the child checks to be sure all is well, goes back to sleep, and generally doesn't remember this waking in the morning. Sometimes when he wakes during these 'arousals' he has difficulty returning to sleep. *This is a common cause of frequent waking.* If he needs your help to get back to sleep, he will wake you.

It is during this block of time (in the *REM* episodes) that nightmares occur. If he comes to a full waking while moving in and out of the dreaming states, he might be afraid to fall asleep again.

Near morning he returns to another period of deep, non-*REM* sleep. Following another arousal comes another, more intense, *REM* dream episode. After more light sleep and dreaming transitions, he wakes for the day. If the child wakes fully during any of these transitions, he might decide that night is over; he then becomes an *early waker*. If you decide to wake him (to fit your schedule or in an attempt to alter his) during his period of deep sleep, you will both be left out of sorts.

In Practical Terms

As we've seen, sleeping through the night is not as simple or common as we might assume.

- Arousals during the night are normal and need not cause problems.

- Sleep problems can arise when a child cannot put himself back to sleep after the arousals.
- It may be harder for children to sleep undisturbed because a child goes more rapidly through the sleep cycles than an adult; there are more periods of arousals and therefore more chances to awaken.
- Deep sleep occurs early in the night and again for a short while near morning. Sleep terrors are likely to happen at this time.
- Light sleep and dreaming occur in the remainder of the night. Nightmares (vs. sleep terrors) happen during that time.
- You can determine your child's sleep state by her sleep behaviour and by what time she went to sleep.
- This information will help you assess the nature of the sleep disturbance and what your response will be.

Biological Rhythms

All people have biological cycles that govern their days and nights. Called 'Circadian Rhythms', these rhythms include sleeping, waking, hunger, and changes in body temperature

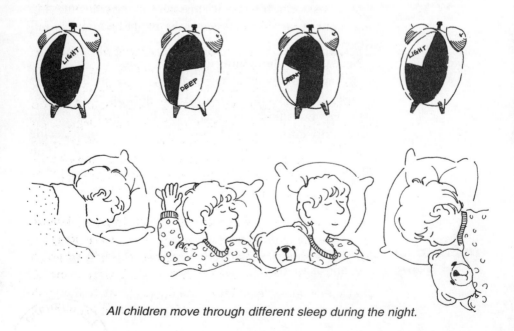

All children move through different sleep during the night.

EXERCISE 2.1: My Child's Sleep Cycle

Using the simplified chart below, superimpose your child's pattern by filling in her bedtime, falling asleep, and waking times. Then add any other night-time occurrences: dreaming, waking, feeding, visits to your room, etc. Make notes about his or her behaviour during those times and compare it to what would be expected during the sleep state. Try to determine what her different states are and how they might be affecting her sleep.

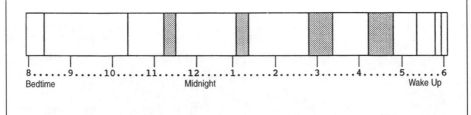

---

and hormones throughout the 24-hour day.[1] The timing of these cycles is linked to the ability to fall and stay asleep. For instance, as we fall asleep there is a drop in our body temperature. We wake up as it starts to rise again.

Research shows that there is a natural tendency to stretch toward a 25-hour cycle. Events in our daytime schedules – mealtime, bedtime, and time of rising – serve the purpose of re-setting the cycle to fit the 24-hour day. You can probably see this happening, to a small degree, on Monday morning after you allowed yourself to go off your usual schedule during the weekend. This is also the experience of 'jet lag' – when the events you experience don't fit with your biological clock.

Most people don't have trouble maintaining a 24-hour cycle. But for children whose sleep cycles have strayed, this is asking a lot. Sometimes we ask children to go to sleep when their bodies are not ready for the sleep cycle. A child would understandably be grumpy and hard to live with if his rhythms were not in sync with the clock of his world.

John just can't seem to get to bed at a decent hour – we always battle at bedtime. When he was eleven months old he wasn't ready to go to bed until 11:00 p.m. We gradually got it down to 9:00 p.m. Then at a year and a half, we noticed it had crept back up to 10:00 p.m.

Biological rhythms influence sleep in several ways.

- It may be necessary to purposefully *take control* of your child's sleep habits if they have got out of kilter.
- Daytime routines are important to maintain biological rhythms and the resulting sense of well-being.
- If you implicate biological rhythms as a part of your child's sleep problems, changes need to be made in *gradual increments* so that a shift of body cycles can occur smoothly.
- When your child is sleeping better and more regularly, you can expect a happier child.

Sleep Associations

The conditions present while going to sleep are called 'sleep associations'.[2] They are the things, events, people, and anything else that might surround or induce sleep.

We all tend to look forward to, and even depend on, the same, or at least a similar set of sleep conditions being there for us each time we want to fall asleep. These are different and personal for each of us. They usually include things like a dark room, a favourite side of the bed, or that special pillow.

Sleep associations help us get to sleep. Routines and rituals are an important part of most people's lives – but nowhere are they more common, and more important, than when they centre around sleep. They seem to help bridge the gap between day and night, wakeful activity and the unknowns of sleep. Even as adults – logical, rational, and usually wanting *more* sleep – we go through certain steps to be sure everything is 'right' for sleep.

I can't go to sleep without reading for a while.

I set a glass of water on the bedside table, plump up my pillow, check the alarm twice, and then relax.

Children learn to go to sleep in the conditions that their parents set up. They learn to expect that old blanket, the night light, the music box, or their special pillow.

Kevin was always rocked to sleep. We made sure that he was fast asleep when we laid him down; otherwise he would cry. If he woke up later, he would cry until we rocked him again.

Since adults are generally in charge of their own lives, they are, theoretically, also in charge of their own sleeping conditions. Imagine what would happen if they were not. Suppose that the parent noted above, when awakened by a windstorm, was all out of water – or, worse yet, discovered someone had hidden her alarm clock. How could she possibly get back to sleep worrying that she might not wake up on time?

Children often find themselves in such frustrating situations. They wake during the night to find that the *conditions they went to sleep with somehow changed during the night.*

Remember that arousals are a normal part of sleep cycles – a time when we check to be sure everything is as it should be before we fall back to sleep. How lonely a child who has fallen asleep at the breast must feel to discover that it is no longer nearby! The bed must certainly feel less comfortable than Daddy's arms or the rocking chair. Certainly calling out or crying is a logical, understandable, reaction – an attempt to regain the conditions favourable to sleep.

Difficulty falling asleep and frequent waking are common sleep problems. They may be connected. When a child cannot *get* to sleep, he will also not be able to get *back* to sleep. His sleep associations can be the root of it all. Even if you do not suspect this to be your child's problem, it is important to look at it. Developing independent sleep associations is also a preventive measure. We will look at prevention more, later in this chapter.

Exercise 2.2 will help you to look at the set of circumstances your child expects and needs in order to fall asleep.

EXERCISE 2.2: Determining Your Child's Sleep Associations

Describe your usual bedtime routine:

What events precede bedtime? (Examples: give bath, put on pyjamas, quiet play, put baby into bed, sing lullaby, turn down lights, say goodnight, leave the room.)

Describe the sleep environment. (Examples: lights low, child in own bed, stuffed bear, blanket in bed.)

Who takes the active parts? (Examples: Dad does quiet play, Mum puts child in bed.)

Describe your middle of the night response:

What happens when the child wakes up? (Examples: he cries, he comes to our room.)

What is the child needing from you? What do you do in response? (Examples: feed him, give her the dummy, scold her, etc.)

Who takes the active parts? (Examples: Dad calls back to her, Mum nurses, etc.)

Assess your child's sleep associations:

From your answers above, summarize the set of circumstances that your child seems to need and expect to get to sleep – the things that signal to her that all is okay and it's time to go to sleep.

Sleep Needs and Patterns

The purpose of looking at norms is not to say that all children have the same needs and can be neatly categorized. Because you are reading this book, it is safe to assume that your child does not fit the pattern outlined. It is also safe to say that you are not pleased and you sense something is going wrong. The purpose of this section is *not* to make you feel worse about yourself or your child.

Norms are very useful to pinpoint problem areas – to help you establish where you are now. Using the norms, you can begin to look at your situation realistically. You will have something to compare your experience to besides, 'When you were a child . . .' and 'None of my children . . .'.

Norms are also useful in setting realistic goals. When the problem is solved you will have clear comparisons for determining how far you have come. Read this section with these thoughts in mind.

Typical Sleep Patterns

Typical sleep patterns vary with the age of the child; we will look at the typical patterns from birth to six years.

Newborns. The first six to eight weeks are called 'unsettled'. During this time, sleeping and eating patterns are not very predictable. A healthy newborn sleeps about sixteen or seventeen hours a day. This occurs during about seven periods throughout the day and night.

By the age of three or four months an infant sleeps about fifteen hours a day. Sleep occurs in about four or five periods. Approximately two-thirds of her sleep is at night. This is what sleep research defines as 'settled' – that is, she sleeps from a late night feeding to an early morning one.

Six Months. By six months, night-time sleep has increased to about twelve hours at night with some possible, occasional, brief wakings. She will also take two naps a day (mid-morning and mid-afternoon), each nap about one to two hours long.

Babies settle in various ways. Some children simply sleep through a feeding. Others gradually push the feeding later and later. Others are unpredictable. However, somewhere between three to six months a baby can sleep a long stretch at night.

One Year. Fourteen hours of sleep is typical for most one-year-olds. If some of this amount is during a morning nap, you can expect her to give that up sometime during the second year.

Two to Six Years. Refer to Table 2.2 *Average Sleep Needs*. Note that the afternoon nap disappears somewhere between three and four years.

A Word About Babies

Sleep disturbances are common with babies. They are so common that many parents are reluctant to define their situation as a 'problem'.

TABLE 2.2: Average Sleep Needs

This table lists the average sleep needs of children from one week old to six years of age. The sleep needs are divided into daytime (naps) and night-time. The night-time averages are represented by the dark coloured bar, and the daytime averages are represented by the light coloured bar. Remember, these are average needs and individual children's needs will vary.

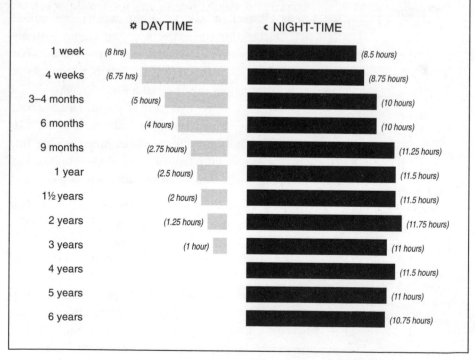

	✿ DAYTIME	‹ NIGHT-TIME
1 week	(8 hrs)	(8.5 hours)
4 weeks	(6.75 hrs)	(8.75 hours)
3–4 months	(5 hours)	(10 hours)
6 months	(4 hours)	(10 hours)
9 months	(2.75 hours)	(11.25 hours)
1 year	(2.5 hours)	(11.5 hours)
1½ years	(2 hours)	(11.5 hours)
2 years	(1.25 hours)	(11.75 hours)
3 years	(1 hour)	(11 hours)
4 years		(11.5 hours)
5 years		(11 hours)
6 years		(10.75 hours)

A baby seems to change every day; as she grows and learns, parents expect that she will learn to sleep when she is able. Some babies learn on their own. Some do not. The advantage of working on sleep problems with infants is that their habits are not as ingrained. Sometimes by making a small change, a parent can bring about a real improvement. Things may improve on their own if you wait long enough, but you may not be able to wait. Or things could get worse

---

EXERCISE 2.3: My Child's Sleep History

Look at your child's sleep patterns over his lifetime. This will give you a sense of problems that persist and problems that change. This is a three-part exercise.

Part 1. Try to remember your child's sleep patterns since birth. Using the form below, place an X in the column that best fits his style of sleep at each age. If there were significant issues at ages not listed, be sure to alter the ages and issues to fit your child.

Part 2. Write a brief description of the behaviour he showed (e.g. 'feeding every two hours around the clock' or 'irregular naps').

Part 3. Note whether the problem cleared up by itself, was resolved after you intervened, or still exists.

ISSUE	6–8 wks	3–4 mo's	6 mo's	18 mo's	2 yrs	3 yrs	4 yrs	5 yrs	6 yrs
unpredictable sleep									
no more night feedings									
sleeps eight-hour stretch									
day naps unpredictable									
middle of night waking									
wakes frightened									
wanders in sleep									
illness									
needs parent									
baulks at bedtime									
wakes too early									
unexplained waking									
other									

and harder to change. If your infant is six months or older, now is a good time to begin.

Will feeding solid food early help my child sleep better? Research does not support this idea. Sleeping a long stretch at night has more to do with neurological than with digestive functioning. The current medical recommendation is to start solid food at four to six months of age. Your child's doctor can help you determine the best time for your child according to his size, birth weight, and health.

It probably will not hurt to try offering solids, but do not hope for instant success. Also, remember that over-feeding at bedtime will only lead to disrupted sleep. Try to avoid 'stuffing' him right before bed.

There are ways that feeding can be used to affect sleep. Mealtime is one of the factors that helps to re-set the internal time clock. Making meals as regular as possible during the day helps give rhythm to a child's day and night. When working to change a skewed schedule, moving the mealtime helps establish a new beginning or ending to the day. Solid food at predictable, longer intervals during the day can help lengthen time between meals at day and *night*. Offering a solid food snack after the last nursing can help prevent falling asleep at the bottle or breast.

In summary, food will not necessarily 'keep him full' through the night, but it can be used to cue him for sleep.

Reasons for Difficult Sleep

Sleep patterns are continually changing because any of the things that affect a child during the daytime can also affect his sleep. This means that there are times in your child's life when you might expect his sleep to be affected. Examples could be: teething, illness, the arrival of a new baby, seasonal changes, or dreaming.

After the cause of such a disturbance is addressed, some children slip back naturally into smooth sleep patterns. Others learn new habits or are thrown into such disequilibrium that the wakefulness continues. This may be the beginning of sleep difficulties. *Recognizing the changes as they occur can help you keep watch to see if a desirable pattern is developing.*

TABLE 2.3: Ways Normal Development Affects Sleep

Age	Possible Sleep Changes	Suggestions
4–5 months	Aware of differences between people; cries when put down.	Begin teaching her to sleep in own bed. Comfort her there with patting, rubbing – work toward laying her down and leaving.
	Wants to touch everything; easily distracted. Rolls over.	Remove excess stimulation (cot toys). Don't assume, that because she balks, she isn't tired. Flip her back over and leave. Encourage rolling both ways during the day. Be patient (and minimally involved) until she learns. Teach her to sleep in various positions.
5–7 months	Creeps/crawls; won't lie still when put down.	Use slow, calming routine to wind down. Allow her to move about until she feels comfortable – but don't expect her to fall asleep immediately.
8–12 months	Good sleepers may now begin to wake at night.	Common time for sleep problems to develop. Make your response as matter-of-fact as possible. Avoid reinforcing the waking (so as to prevent new habits from forming).
	Separation issues peak.	Probably not a good time to cry-it-out alone (crying may just escalate). Pop back in at bedtime – make visits brief; try not to pick her up. Encourage use of favourite blanket, toy, or 'lovey'.
Toddler to 3 yrs	Separation issues again.	Respond as above.
	Fears are strong – may seem irrational.	Respond as for separation issues. Stay calm and reassuring. Alter sleeping environment as needed (door open, light on, etc.)
	Negative, power struggles; resists sleep and naps.	Try not to engage in battle. Instead, stay calm and matter-of-fact.
	Refuses comfort from one parent.	Don't take it personally. Share or alternate sleep duty. Be more involved in other activities (bath, play). It will pass. Try again when you sense less negativism.
Pre-school 3–5 yrs	Excited about life; physically active; procrastinates at bedtime; climbs out of bed.	Keep play before bed calm. Expect a lengthy bedtime routine. Decide on limits in advance.
	Imagination expands; fears and nightmares emerge; wants you present at bedtime and during night.	Decide on strategy in advance, according to family values. Teach coping skills during the day.
	Expresses independence; wants to extend bedtime; may fight naptime.	Try not to engage in battle. Ask her wishes and incorporate them into sleep routine. Where possible, find other areas of life in which to empower her.

You can decide how long to allow a child to re-establish a desirable pattern on his own. Several factors should be taken into consideration:

- His history of being able to settle himself: after his last illness, did he return quickly to his old patterns or did you need to 'draw the line'?
- His temperament: is he a 'natural night owl' who will take any opportunity to stay awake?
- His needs: how well is he coping during the day with reduced sleep?
- Your needs: how are you coping? How long can you wait it out?

When a reasonable amount of time has passed and you have decided that a new habit has formed or has the potential to develop, you can change your response or intervene with the method that works for you.

Normal Development Affects Sleep

When children make developmental strides, it can send them into disequilibrium – and sleep is disrupted. This can affect a child in several ways.

He may be so excited about learning a new skill that he has a hard time settling down – he may even be driven to practice skills in his sleep. During that normal arousal, instead of going right back to sleep, the new 'stander' stands in his cot. It may be easier to understand if you relate it to yourself: think about a time you were learning a new skill – when you were dreaming about tennis, going over that shot you missed, or worrying about the match the next day.

Mastering one skill brings a child quickly to the next frustration. When she stands in her cot, she may cry desperately because she hasn't yet learned how to get herself down. She needs you to help until she can help herself again. She needs a little extra reassurance, so separation difficulties are common.

Dealing with developmental sleep issues may be particularly frustrating because parents do not have control over a child's development. Sometimes the only 'cure' is allowing the development to continue on its own with

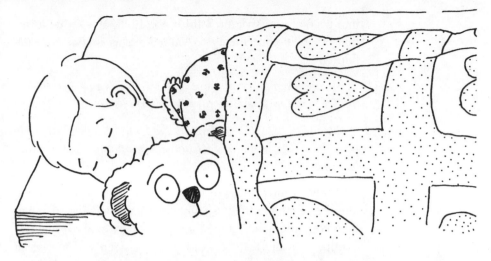

Sleeping like a baby.

encouraging messages from you. It helps to recognize that the transition will probably be short-lived. Overreacting and doing too much can only *prolong* the problem if she becomes dependent upon your help to go to sleep.

Although each child is an individual, there are guidelines and basic information that apply to all. Table 3 summarizes the affect of development on sleep. With this foundation, you can begin to look at the specific issues concerning you about your child.

Tips to Avoid Sleep Problems

If you are expecting your next child, a word about prevention is in order. To begin establishing positive sleep patterns in your child, there are three things to do: Identify your family values, set goals, and be alert to the tendency to veer off course.

Know What You Want   It is much easier to prevent a problem than to solve it. And it is easier to solve a problem if you know what you want.

Values. As you plan for the ideal sleep situation, take into account the specific values you hold, and set expectations that fit your lifestyle. Values are as unique as each family.

We are frequently out evenings, so we value Maureen's ability to get to sleep smoothly – and on her own.

Because my wife works late and enjoys spending time with the kids when she gets home, we appreciate their late bedtimes.

Goals. Your values will clarify the goals toward which to aim. For example, if you value everyone sleeping together, then your goal is to arrange a family bed where everyone is comfortable and teaching independent sleep will not be an issue. If you value independent sleep, you will not take your child into your bed under normal circumstances.

As you carry on, check to be sure your action supports your goal – watch that 'just for tonight' doesn't slip into an unwanted pattern.

Since it is important to us that each child stay in her own room, our goal is to teach independent sleep habits. We'll keep Hannah in our room only the first months.

Be Alert to Pitfalls It is the family who values independent sleep that is most likely to fall off course – usually without even knowing it. If independent sleep is your goal, be alert to the pitfalls.

Sleep Associations (see Chapter 1) are all of the circumstances that surround going to sleep. This includes the setting, timing, aids, and people involved. If you value independent sleep you will want to keep yourselves, your help, or presence, out of the child's sleep associations as much as possible. Make sure the bedtime circumstances stay the same throughout the night so your child can put herself back to sleep without help.

Keeping Sleep Associations Simple A general guideline is to allow an infant about five or six months old to establish her own sleep habits. By then, most children have the neurological maturity to sleep more soundly. When your child is between four and six months old, begin to encourage the sleep associations you value.

The following is a discussion of the sleep associations that most commonly cause problems.

Feeding. The child who is nursed or fed to sleep learns to need the calming that comes from eating, sucking, and being held. If she rouses during the night, she will call for more of the same. She may also wake seeming 'rested' with a burp after 20 minutes, but she will not be establishing dependable routines.

EXERCISE 2.4: Plans for Prevention

The best way to prevent sleep hassles is to look at your values and goals, then make a plan to achieve those goals.

Values: Decide what is important to you concerning your child's sleep. Define the ideal bedtime scenario for the middle of the night, morning, and naptime.

Goals: Determine the goals that will support those values.

Plan: Implement the plan to achieve the goals.

Sample answers.
Values: I enjoy having my children close to me at night. **Or** I don't want a bedtime battle – a nice tucking-in and goodnight should do it. **Goals:** Child learns to sleep with parent nearby, probably in parental or family bed. **Or** Child learns to fall asleep easily, on his own. **Plan:** Welcome him in parental bed from birth until he asks to sleep elsewhere. **Or** Put him in bed to fall asleep. Allow him to cry if need be.

As she loses that newborn drowsiness, begin to keep her awake during feedings (easier said than done for some babies) or purposely rouse her while laying her down so that she knows she is falling asleep in her own bed, not in your arms.

Sucking. Dummies help some children settle themselves to sleep. Be aware that their use after about three or four months means that this habit will eventually need to be unlearned.

Rocking. Rocking is a pleasant, calming experience for both child and parent, but it can be a *strong* sleep association. One alternative is to rock a child to soothe and lull him, but not put him into a full sleep. Or rock until it ceases to be soothing – perhaps at four or five months with the sociable child, or later, as mobility increases, when she squirms to get down to play.

Children love to 'nest' – that is, move around in bed until

EXERCISE 2.5: Simplify Sleep Associations

1. List or describe the circumstances that presently surround your child at sleep-time:

2. Place a check by those that might get in the way of your ultimate goal.

3. Circle those that you might try to eliminate – or begin working on – at this time.

4. Make special note of those that need to stay in place now but might cause problems later.

it feels just right. If we confine them by rocking, walking, or whatever, we deny them this winding down pleasure. If you are a 'pillow fluffer' yourself, you will understand.

Loveys. Many children become attached to special blankets, stuffed animals or toys. 'Loveys' make it easier to sleep without parents. To avoid the panic of a lost or forgotten lovey, make more than one available (buy matching blankets) or make it so general that a replacement might not be noticed.

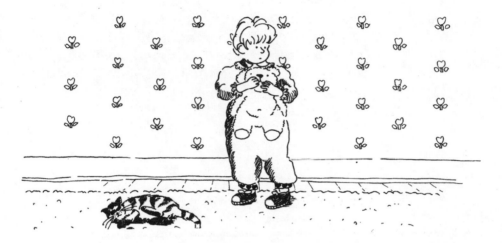

Loveys can be there when you're not.

Summary

In summary, keep the sleep setting as simple as possible. It needs to stay the same all night – so he will not wake up confused or angry when the place he went to sleep has changed, or people are nowhere to be seen. Keep parental involvement as minimal as possible except for special circumstances. He makes the decision about what works best for him within the structure you have provided.

Establishing the sleep patterns you value may prevent sleep from becoming an issue. Patterns change as children grow and change. Having learned a 'solid base' will give you and your child a standard to refer to; it is much easier to *re-learn* than to change long-standing habits.

Additional *Solve Your Child's Sleep Problems* by Richard Ferber, M.D.
Reading Dorling Kindersley, London, 1986.

Healthy Sleep Habits, Happy Child by Marc Weissbluth,
M.D. Fawcett Columbine, New York, 1987. UK distributor:
Tiptree Book Services, Tiptree, Colchester CO5 0SR.

Chapter 3   THE TROUBLE SPOTS

Is there a time of day or night that you dread? Maybe it's the fight at naptime, or that first early morning call, or the inevitable middle-of-the-night visit.

Take a minute to look at your trouble spots. Certainly a child can show more than one problem at more than one time of day, but the first step is to figure out 'what is happening when?' In this chapter we will break down the day into segments where sleep is likely to become an issue. There are new ways to think about things and some tips to try. Some ideas apply primarily to infants, others are more applicable to older children. Feel free to focus on what fits your child and family the most.

Separation Anxieties

To fall asleep means to be separated from those you love and trust. It is no casy task and is especially hard during times of developmental upheaval. Sleep problems often show themselves when separation anxieties are an expected part of development. A child might think the following:

When I close my eyes, it's dark – everything is gone. I wonder where I am going . . . and I wonder where you are.

A parent's job is to find the balance between being supportive and being firm, to be sure in her own heart that nothing bad will happen to the child while he sleeps – then to communicate that in a cheerful, confident manner.

Let him borrow some of your confidence until he develops his own. Reassure him you are nearby. Call to him or visit occasionally if that helps. Tell him what you do while he sleeps (something boring). After rest time, point out that he woke safely and you were there.

Dr Spock recommends that parents of children who are experiencing peak separation issues sit in a chair next to their beds until they fall asleep. Don't over-coddle, but don't

39

abandon him to tough it out on his own. Because he really needs to see you, letting him cry-it-out at peak separation times will only escalate the fear and crying.

The Importance of Rituals

The purpose of a bedtime ritual is two-fold. First, it eases that transition from wakefulness to sleep and, in many cases, to being alone. Second, it signals him 'time to go to sleep' or 'it's okay to go back to sleep'.

To fulfil its purpose, the ritual needs to have certain characteristics. It needs to be calming – reading and singing vs. active or imaginary play – and reassuring for him.

I talk in a soothing voice about how much fun we had during the day, how proud Grandma is of her, how exciting it is to see her explore everything. Maybe she doesn't understand everything I say yet, but I know she gets the loving message from me.

The ritual needs to become routine and be very similar for every bedtime. There is no need to be rigid – just consistent. Ideally, it can be carried out by anyone so that it remains a comfort rather than a stress if another parent or sitter puts the child to bed.

I was annoyed because my husband wouldn't sing 'Rock-a-bye-baby' to Amy when he put her to sleep. After all, that's the way I did it, and she seemed to need it. Then I changed my strategy and my song, too. Now Amy expects a song, but it can be any song, sung by anyone – so now we can trade off bedtime duty!

The ritual should be just long enough to ease the transition, not to get the child to sleep. If it is simple, it will not become a burden. If it is too long, your own discomfort with leaving your child may be transferred. If you remain in the room until he gets to sleep, then he becomes dependent on your presence to get to – and back to – sleep.

I show him his cot and try to convey my good feelings about it so that he will see his bed as his special place. We say goodnight to his bear. I lay him down with his blanket.

Saying 'night-night' and turning down the light is his cue that I am leaving.

Rituals are not set in stone, but will change as the child grows and his needs change. When life seems out of control, returning to a ritual might be just what is needed.

Transitional Objects

Attachment to a special object is a healthy way to deal with fears. 'Transitional objects' bridge the gap between parent and child – the gap that is a sign of blossoming independence. Reality is that Mum and Dad can't always be there, but other self-comforting things can be. Often called 'loveys', these items can be nearly anything – a special blanket or a special toy – that the child is attached to. Dr T. Berry Brazelton, author of *To Listen to a Child*, emphasizes that the use of a 'lovey' is key in encouraging independent sleep.[1]

The child who doesn't spontaneously form such an attachment can be encouraged to do so. The parent chooses something and places it with the child at bedtime and other happy or stressful times during the day. Use a phrase such as, 'Bear is here to hug you and keep you company.'

Don't be concerned if the attachment continues through the preschool years or longer. Learning to make attachments is one of the primary goals of childhood.

Getting Mobile Kids Into Bed

One challenge most parents face is making bedtime pleasant for the older toddler and preschooler. You probably want her to sleep more than she does. For her, bedtime or naptime is an invasion of her time. Remember that a child's play is her 'work'. Imagine how you would feel if someone told you to go to bed when you had just put a cake in the oven or had just sat down with some important clients.

A 'five-minute warning' gives her time to wind down or finish up. It gives her the sense that you respect what she is doing, but that you also respect the bedtime you've set for her.

Attachment objects are still very important to the older child. Even though she looks grown up, you needn't fear that she is 'being a baby' if she still wants her teddy bear or blanket. Incorporate it into your routine.

Routines continue to be meaningful. An astute pre-schooler can be a master at procrastination – one story easily leads to two or three. If part of the bedtime ritual that she looks forward to occurs *in* bed, getting her there is not as troublesome.

When we read to him on the couch, it is amazing how many hassles come up on the short walk from the living room to his bedroom. When we read in his bed, he becomes drowsy – right where we want him to be.

Reading is an experience that **children often enjoy as part of the bedtime routine**. Older preschoolers can be introduced to 'chapter books'. Looking forward to what will happen next is a reason to get ready for bed.

The quiet time alone with Mum or Dad at the end of the day may be enough of a lure in and of itself. If the time is full of threats or spankings, he begins to expect a negative bedtime, and his behaviour might deteriorate in anticipation of the struggle.

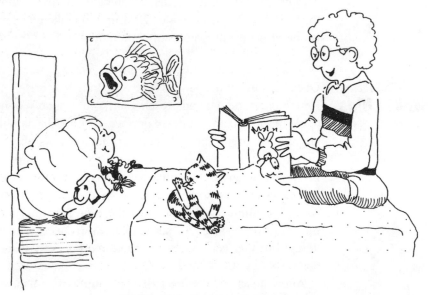

Stories make bedtime more fun.

Keeping Kids in Bed

As children grow older, there are no more cot rails to contain the resistant sleeper! The night waker becomes the night walker, and parents can feel powerless. Here are several ideas to try to keep kids in bed.

If possible, prevention is the best tactic. This may involve a little work on your part to be ready to respond to a request by going *to* her. You decide how many glasses of water you bring before firmly announcing that this is your last. Setting limits calmly, without anger, is less likely to bring out resistance.

Say more than one 'goodnight'. It takes some children a long time to fall asleep. Promise that you will return to check on her in five minutes – then do! Check just before you sense she is ready to climb out so you reward her staying in bed. Return several times if you need to – extending the time in your own mind. Once she actually lays still, she may fall asleep. If she does, tell her in the morning that you checked on her and gave her a kiss. Just be sure she isn't keeping herself up for your next visit.

You might find some 'work' to do down the hall or even in her room – stay nearby but don't make an issue of it.

Some children talk about feeling alone and lonely. Even after they know you still 'exist', emotionally they just want to be with you. It may help to leave a little part of Mum or Dad with the child – Dad's shoes near the door, Mum's sweater at the foot of the bed. How about company in the form of a turtle, a goldfish – or even a sibling?

We thought that sharing a room would keep the kids awake, but it did just the opposite. Oh, they giggle a while, so bedtime's later, but they seem to feel better knowing they aren't alone.

Children age three and a half and older often respond to a reward system. It can be as simple as a special breakfast for staying in bed and sleeping all night long. It can be in the form of a chart where the child earns a star (and a hug) for each night of staying in bed. A trouble-filled night should not be reinforced with threats or scolding – just with the absence of the star and with a message that tomorrow will be better and will certainly earn a new star. When your child takes an active part in the planning, he will be more invested in cooperating.

Some people need a winding-down time before falling asleep. How many adults do you know who read themselves to sleep? The same tactic can work for children. Your child can take a certain number of books to bed with her. Or she can be given a length of time for reading before 'lights out' or before the second and final tucking-in. Music can be used the same way.

When prevention doesn't work, you need to step up your programme. Sometimes, no matter how many creative plans you devise, your child keeps hopping out of bed – laughing or crying piteously, taunting your sense of control. He may wander the house at night or come into your bedroom. Safety becomes a concern. Locking the door is not advisable because of emotional and safety factors (for example, in case of fire). A locked door adds to the child's fear – it is hard to work on learning to stay alone when one is feeling fearful. A 'baby gate' suggests that he needs to stay in his room; however, adventuresome kids can easily hop over one. Two safety gates placed one above the other are harder to get out of, but he can still look out and you can look in. He might react with anger. Experiment a little – remembering to give each idea a reasonable amount of time.

If you can remain calm, try the 'Endurance Challenge'. Calmly lead the child back to his bed – as many times as necessary. Avoid eye contact. Do not talk except to repeat the same simple phrase, such as, 'It's time to go to sleep.'

I kept telling myself that I was the adult and I could outlast him. I returned him 52 times the first night. By the third night he got tired of the game and knew I wasn't going to give up.

This will not be easy, but it will pay off. A similar approach is the 'Door-Closing Technique' where the child is given a choice about whether the bedroom door will remain open. (For the child who wants to be with you, having the door open is the next best thing.) If he stays in bed, it remains open; if he gets out it will be shut. A very persistent child will pull or pound on the door – this may escalate before it gets better.

This technique takes a great deal of determination and confidence on the parent's part. Consistency is very important. The book *Solve Your Child's Sleep Problems* (see suggested readings at the end of this chapter) gives a more detailed programme for those families needing a full-scaled approach.

Getting Kids to Sleep

Sometimes trying the tips already mentioned will help the child develop his own way of falling asleep. Other children need a more overall approach in order to learn the skill. These are outlined in Chapter 4 along with guidelines to decide which is most appropriate for your situation.

Late Sleep Cycles

The 'Night Owl' pushes his bedtime later and later. His internal clock needs to be gradually reset. Be sure there is nothing during the day that encourages late bedtime (for example, a late nap or dinner). If you are currently battling, defuse the battle awhile by letting him keep the late bedtime for now.

Since you can't *make* someone go to sleep, begin making changes in the morning. Wake him the same time each morning. Reset any other events that might be off – for example, move mealtimes.

Begin moving his bedtime 15 minutes earlier for a few days, then 15 minutes earlier again as many times as needed until bedtime is more appropriate. Make gradual changes, waiting as long as is necessary for him to adjust before you change again.

It is relatively easy to work on this problem, but watch for its easy return! The natural tendency is to keep pushing bedtime later.

Occasionally there are children who require substantially less (or more) sleep than is the norm. Check with a physician to rule out any physical causes. If the child's daytime functioning in not impaired, learning to live with it may be a good tactic. See Chapter 4 for more related information; safety and sharing 'awake' duty are two issues to consider.

Night Fears   For a child, going to sleep means being totally vulnerable, away from the people who keep him safe. Normal fears are exaggerated at night. Sleeping with the light on or door open will disturb his sleep far less than will his fears.

Fears are not usually clearly stated, but can be seen in the reluctance to separate. If your bedtime ritual includes some discussion about things you plan to do tomorrow – for example, what is for breakfast – you make it clear that life goes on.

Middle of the Night. Assess your middle-of-the-night reaction. Be sure you are involved as little as possible, and that your action is not rewarding or subtly reinforcing your child's waking. Exercise 3.1 will help you think this through.

Hunger and Night Feeders   *She is still waking every couple of hours for feeding . . . I'm exhausted! Will it ever stop?*

That question is probably best answered by gathering information from several sources, then weighing it against your own opinions, instincts, and need for sleep. Ask your doctor whether your child has a nutritional need for night feedings. Ask yourself whether she has other needs met by night feedings, and ask whether these needs could be met in other ways.

EXERCISE 3.1: Night-time Rewards

Learning theory states that people tend to repeat actions for which they are rewarded; they hope they will be rewarded again. When a child feels his night waking is rewarded (i.e. he gets something) he continues to wake. Here is a list of typical middle-of-the-night responses. Number in order what you suspect is the least to the most rewarding for your child.

_____ feeding	_____ patting
_____ giving drink of water	_____ taking to parental bed
_____ rocking	_____ calling out from your room
_____ walking	_____ discipline

Only you can define it as a 'problem'. If your child is considerably past three or four months and still requiring frequent night feedings, you might want to re-think your situation.

Feeding becomes a problem when eating or sucking is the condition necessary to bring on sleep. Remember that arousals during the night are normal. If suckling gets the child to sleep, she will cry after waking for someone to bring back that sucking condition so she can get back to sleep.

She cries and cries – really demanding to be fed. Sure enough, when I do feed her she eats ravenously and then falls back to sleep.

Sucking and eating also serve a comforting function. If you feel comfortable using feedings for this purpose and you do not feel it is influencing sleep patterns, then you will not perceive it as a problem.

If you look at your own eating patterns, you will see that we all feel hungry at times when we are used to eating. Similarly, children become accustomed to eating several times a night if feedings continue to be offered. It becomes a 'chicken/egg' situation when this 'learned hunger' triggers waking.

There is also some question about whether food itself can cause uncomfortable sleep. Eating keeps the digestive system activated during the time when it is meant to be inactive for the night. To add to the confusion, babies with stomach pains often give the same cues as those who are hungry. More food perpetuates the cycle.

Watch for signs, and experiment with other ways to get your child 'over the hump' of feeding at night.

I continued to feed Sandy every time she woke because it was the quickest way to get us back to sleep. I never questioned it. Then one night I experimented by rubbing her back a little – she went back to sleep. That was my cue that she didn't need food at night. Soon she stopped waking at all.

Snackers These children wake frequently at night for food. Most often they are also daytime snackers who have not learned to go

---

EXERCISE 3.2: How Much Is Too Much?

Instructions: Determine how much milk your child consumes at night.

Breast-feeders: Time the length of nursing (swallowing). If sessions last more than two or three minutes and occur more than one or two times a night, the volume may be excessive for a six-month-old child or older. Soaking wet nappies are also a clue the child may be getting too much milk at night.

Bottle-feeders: Measure the amount of milk drunk at night out of the total daily intake. Compare to suggested norms: a child between the ages of six months and one year drinks approximately 24–32 oz. milk per 24 hour day.
Note: The amount of milk does not increase with age beyond a year because it is supplemented with solid food.

---

long intervals between feedings. They may nurse between solid feedings or sip on bottles during the day.

The problem is tackled during the day by gradually lengthening the time between eating. An infant might be encouraged to go longer between bottles, eat from both breasts, or nurse at solid food times; a toddler can be distracted and entertained to keep him away from bottle-sipping.

When snacking is the issue, night-time wakings may spontaneously decrease when daytime feedings become more regular.

There are several ways you can approach solving the problem of snacking during the night.

Decrease the amount of night food. For bottle feeders you can gradually, progressively dilute the milk with water so that the amount of actual food is decreased. It also becomes unpalatable so the child loses interest.

Or you can fill bottles with a smaller and smaller amount so he becomes accustomed to eating less.

Adjust the night feeding schedule. If you and the paediatrician decide that your child is consuming too much food, too frequently at night, another tactic might be explored. 'Learned' or not, the baby probably is 'hungry'. A hungry baby cannot easily be left unattended since the cry of hunger truly escalates. A 'cold turkey' approach would not be kind. Instead, adjusting the night-time feeding schedule can solve this problem gradually. Consult your GP or your local well baby clinic for help with changing the amounts of food.

Altering your child's sleep habits by adjusting his feeding schedule can be done in two steps.[2] First, eliminate the night feedings and the hunger at inappropriate *times*. Second, teach new ways to get to sleep. You can work on both at the same time if it feels comfortable to you. Or you can continue to offer yourself as comforter for a while since you are making a major change by not offering the expected feeding. Then, after you and baby have passed the first hump, you can teach him to fall asleep on his own.

To eliminate night feedings, decrease the amount of milk in the bottle and increase the time between feedings. That is, give him less food, less often. On the first night, bottles contain one ounce less than usual (or one to two minutes less than his usual nursing time). Feed him at no more than two-hour intervals. Each night, decrease the amount in the bottle by one more ounce. Then increase the minimum amount of time between feedings by a half hour.

When he has finished eating (he may still be awake), lay him down and soothe him to sleep in his bed however you choose. Don't pick him up – this only makes the eating or nursing position available and, since he can't eat, frustrating for him.

He also may wake before the established minimum time has passed. Soothe him in ways that don't involve eating. If you find your actions or presence are not helpful, or even upset him more, leave him to handle it in his own way. Don't give in. Help him to learn to wait.

At the end of the first week, no more food will be offered during the night. If night wakings are not rewarded by food, they may disappear. If he continues to wake but seems to need your help and soothing to get him back to sleep, you can teach him to sleep using the method described in Chapter 4.

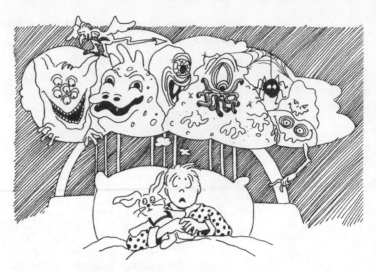

Nightmares are normal for preschoolers.

This is a gradual process. If it is too fast for you, you can make the decreases in the amount of food every other night. Know that it will take a little longer.

Danny was eight months old when I decided to slowly cut back on the amount of formula he got at each waking. As the amount of formula decreased, he seemed a little surprised that the feeding was over so quickly – and before he had gone back to sleep. I had to put him in his bed and rub his back until he dropped off. I could have just let him cry alone, but I figured one major change at a time was enough. My first goal was to get him used to less food, less often.

Since he was pretty set in his night-time schedule, the 'less often' part was harder for me. At first he woke at his regular time expecting a feeding, but we were trying to extend the time between feedings. We found it easier on all of us if my husband did the before-feeding comforting.

One night my husband kept patting and Danny just fell back to sleep. We saw that as a major turning point and no longer offered any food. He still woke, although not as frequently or as desperately, and responded quite quickly to soothing. Before long we just gave a little pat of reassurance and left him alone to fall asleep. Now he seldom calls for us.

Once the basic feeding problem has been solved, learning new sleep habits can be relatively quick.

Nightmares

I had a bad dream . . . can I sleep with you?

Remember that the dream state occurs during the middle and latter part of the night. (See Table 1 in Chapter 2.) Be certain it is a nightmare rather than sleep terror. We will discuss both in this section.

A preschooler with a healthy imagination is hazy about the difference between real and unreal. She needs to be *taught* about dreams. Gearing to her age level, explain that all people have dreams – both good and bad:

Katie, did you know that our imagination works even when we are sleeping? In good dreams your imagination puts you in happy, fun places. You can pretend to be swimming or playing or running – but it's just your imagination. But really, you are still asleep in your bedroom. In bad dreams your imagination puts you in scary, bad places . . . sometimes with scary, bad things or people. It feels very, very real – but it is just your imagination. You are still asleep and safe in your bedroom. When you open your eyes and look around your room, you will see that you are home and safe, and that Mum and Dad are nearby. Then you can go back to sleep.

Teaching is done during the day when the child is calm and receptive – no one is able to learn right after a dream. Do some imagination play together during the day to show the child that she can invent both happy and scary situations – and stay in the bedroom the whole time!

Parents who advocate the Family Bed will welcome the child into their own bed. Other parents may make a special consideration after occasional bad dreams. If you fear this might begin a new habit, return the child to her bed, comfort her, and stay with her until she falls asleep. Be reassuring and share your confidence that her bedroom is a safe place for her to be and that you are always nearby.

A child needs to be prepared for what to do after a bad dream just as with any other special situation (like fire drills or getting lost). Incorporate her ideas about what would be helpful, then practice during the day:

When you have a bad dream, first, turn on the light and look around to see you are in your own room. Find your special bear – snuggle down tight, and go back to sleep. You can even leave the light on in case you want to look around some more.

Don't expect her to carry it out on her own. When she is frightened, she won't be rational. After a dream, you go through the steps with her – this adds predictability to her night and helps her gain self-confidence.

Nightmares are quite normal. Sometimes you can relate them to upsetting thoughts or events. Or you may never know the cause and the dreams will end as quickly as they began. If your child is truly panicked and terrified, do some serious investigating of the cause and seek professional help.

If you had been working on other sleep problems when the dreams began, expect some regression. In order to not lose all your ground, try not to give in completely. Try some of the suggestions – recognize her feelings, but don't dwell on them.

Sleep Terrors

Josh wakes us up with his screams. His eyes are wide open, but he doesn't seem to see us. He sweats and thrashes around. Nothing we do seems to help. It can happen up to three or four times a week, but he doesn't remember any of it in the morning.

To understand sleep terrors, we need to review our knowledge about sleep cycles. After an hour or so of deep sleep, a child has a brief arousal to lighter sleep and may actually wake. Then comes a second period of deep sleep, followed by another arousal. (There is another deep sleep cycle again before waking in the morning, but it is not usually as deep.)

Generally, the transition between cycles happens quickly and without incident. For some children, the transitions do not happen smoothly. Sometimes they take longer than usual. It is as if, for a while, he is both asleep *and* awake. He can show a range of behaviours from brief eye opening, mumbling, and even sleep walking, to more agitated thrashing, screaming, or appearing to run away. It can be brief or last from about 10 minutes up to an hour. The behaviour subsides when he moves back into the next sleep cycle. In the morning (or at the time, if he wakes fully) he will not remember the incident.

There are no simple explanations as to why only some children are affected, but it seems to be a function of the neurological system. Insufficient sleep and over stimulation can make sleep terrors more likely.

Sleep terrors are said to be most common for three- to four-year-olds. But they probably also occur in younger children, even infants. For children up to five and six, these episodes are part of the normally developing and maturing sleep stages. Because deep sleep is *so* deep for young children, it may be that it is harder for them to make a smooth transition into REM sleep.

Most often, the best solution is to wait for maturation. If sleep terrors continue for the older child, they may have different causes and should be discussed with your doctor.

It is important to distinguish between sleep terrors and nightmares because you deal with each quite differently. Two characteristics to watch for:

- Sleep terrors are not related to dreaming. They most often occur during the first four hours after bedtime. Dreaming doesn't occur until later in the night and early morning.
- When in sleep terror, the child does not seem to be aware of or calmed by your presence. Even though his eyes may be open and he is out of bed, he is not awake. He may act frightened, scream, talk, thrash, or pull away.

To help understand the difference, try Exercise 3.3.

Handling Sleep Terrors

Your instinct will be to make him feel better and to help the incident stop. However, in this case, the less you do, the better. He needs to move through the process until it is over. Even offering comfort can prolong the incident.

EXERCISE 3.3: Distinguishing Nightmares From Sleep Terrors

The following is a list of various night-time behaviours. Mark each with 'N' for Nightmare or 'T' for Terror. Some may fit under both, but the defining behaviours will fit only in one place:

_____ 1. Talks about the witches in her dream.

_____ 2. Screams and cries.

_____ 3. Falls out of bed.

_____ 4. Runs to your room.

_____ 5. Can't settle back down to sleep.

_____ 6. Cries out at 10:00 p.m.

_____ 7. Talks gibberish.

_____ 8. Pushes you away.

_____ 9. Can't remember the distress in the morning.

_____ 10. Is afraid to go to sleep the next night.

_____ 11. Cries out at 2:00 a.m.

Circle the night behaviours in your child that concern you. This will help you determine which type of disturbance your child is experiencing.

Key: Nightmares: 1, 5, 10, 11   Sleep Terrors: 6, 7, 8, 9   Both: 2, 3, 4

Instead of trying to interact with him, try to stand back and watch. Make provisions for his safety, if needed. If he welcomes your comfort, give it. But if he pushes you away, do not feel angry or guilty. He doesn't know what he is doing; his sleep terror is not anything you have caused.

Waking him up would be very difficult – and if you did, he would be confused and frightened. This is where terrors might become confused with nightmares. When questioned, he may invent something he was dreaming about or he may remember the incident in the morning with fear and reluctance to go to bed the next night. Do not share your anxiety with him.

The most important thing you can do is help him get as much rest as possible. Well-rested children have smoother sleep cycles. Excess need for sleep makes moving in and out of the normal sleep cycles more difficult and may result in the confused state of partial waking. Keep a regular daytime routine, especially including naps.

It seems to happen when we have been away from home all day. Billy has been charming and playing happily. I expect him to be so tired that he will conk out all night. Instead, he wakes up shortly after he has gone to sleep, screaming, as if he were in pain. He rolls around and then falls back to sleep.

Sleep terrors are more disturbing for parents than for the child. He will literally sleep right through it, while you remain shaken. The hardest part may be to know that the best help is no help at all. No one likes to be pushed away when offering comfort.

Some children have sleep terrors only occasionally. Others have them for stretches at a time, then go without. Some children experience them once a night, others several times a night. The episodes can vary in intensity and length. Handling them as suggested usually results in a decrease of intensity and frequency. Occasionally there is a child who simply continues having sleep terrors as part of his sleep pattern; parents learn to live with it. Most children outgrow them.

If you are concerned about your child's safety or health, or if you are bothered by the intensity or any other aspect of the episodes, please check with your child's doctor. This has been a brief summary of the very complex subject of sleep terrors. It is intended to alert you to a possible explanation of your child's night-time behaviour.

Early Risers

It is not unusual for an infant to wake around 5:00 or 6:00 a.m. If it is brief, for a feeding or changing, you need not worry.

For an older child, look at what she 'gets' for waking up early: watching early TV shows, crawling in with Mum and Dad, spending time with a parent before work, etc. If the early waking is not rewarded, it may go away.

An early sleep cycle is harder to change than a late one. Interestingly enough, sometimes an *earlier* bedtime makes for more restful sleep. Then the child is more likely to move smoothly through that last morning arousal (transition between sleep states) without waking fully.

Look at the child's daytime schedule and make it as dependable as possible. If the child naps, establish a regular time for it (usually around 1:00 p.m. – and not later than 3:00 p.m.) waking her, if need be. Food and mealtimes can sometimes be used to alter the child's internal clock. A bedtime snack may help postpone an early breakfast.

Early rising is often a discouraging problem – and not easy to solve since you have little control. It often stems from temperament and natural rhythms so the child doesn't have much control over it either.

If the rising time is not too extreme, you might choose to 'live with it'. Pull the baby into bed with you while you doze, or sneak safe toys into her cot after she is asleep to encourage quiet morning play. Leave out a snack for an older child. Childproof the older child's room, then be sure he stays in it. A word of hope: your 'morning lark' may later be easier to get ready for school than her counterpart, the 'night owl'.

Daytime Schedules Affect Night

Children with night-time sleep problems generally appear raring-to-go during the day, but having problems only at night. Parents are surprised when the daytime schedule is the culprit.

As discussed in Chapter 1, our bodies are governed by physiological rhythms. Our internal time clocks are set by the events during the day. Rhythms during the day affect rhythms during the night. Children with sleep problems need stable daytime schedules to prepare their bodies for sleep.

Certainly, during the time that you are working on making changes, it will pay to keep daytime as routine as possible. Later you can experiment with a degree of flexibility.

Naptime – Your Time

I love Sara's naptime. It is my time – time to rejuvenate myself! I hope she doesn't give up her nap until she is fifteen!

Most children move into a single, early afternoon nap somewhere around age one. Some continue to nap into the kindergarten year. Between ages three and four, most children don't seem to need as much sleep and give up naps.

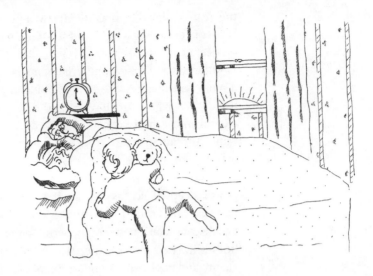

Stable daytime schedules help prevent early rising.

Is it possible to have too much napping time? It is perfectly all right to wake your child after a reasonable amount of time (one to two hours). It is not uncommon for busy toddlers or preschoolers to want a long, late nap (especially when they are working toward giving it up altogether). Bedtime can get pushed later or become a struggle. Especially during times of high activity or new development, a child's inner time clock seems to get out of kilter. You cannot depend on her inner clock making the best decision for her.

Nathan is an absolute bear if I try to wake him up. But he is more pleasant if something wakes him up instead of a person – (me). I begin by making noises near his door – the vacuum cleaner or loud music. I have even been known to stand in the hallway and toss toys onto his bed. He is pleasantly surprised and we make it into a silly game.

This is a time for creativity. Remember, changing someone's internal cycles is a *gradual* process.

Catnaps are trouble makers. It *seems* that a five minute snooze can refresh a child, but it can upset a child's rhythm for the rest of the day and even into the night. Be especially wary of car rides, swings, and feeding times – common catnap inducers.

Often around four months, catnappers work themselves into a more dependable schedule. If you can get your child to fall asleep for a nap in his own bed, the catnap will probably extend into a regular nap. If not, decrease the use of props inducing catnaps and work on getting him used to falling asleep in his own bed.

Some children don't nap easily, or seem to need your help to get to sleep. If so, ask yourself how much time you spend carrying him around. It easily becomes a cycle: you hold him because he won't nap, and he won't nap for long because you hold him. Learn to be alert to the cues when he is getting sleepy and begin encouraging sleep at those times – before he becomes over-tired and into his 'second wind'.

Try not to think of your child as a 'non-napper'. It helps to regulate irregular children by sticking close to routine. Offer the nap time even if it becomes a quiet playtime (learning to play independently for short periods is a skill even babies can practice). Children go through times when naps don't seem very important and they give out signals that they are 'giving up naps'. If you think your child is too young or still needs the rest, don't be too quick to accept the change as permanent.

When nap time becomes a battle, weigh the benefits against the struggle. For those particularly resistant times in a child's life, naptime becomes a prime time to assert himself. Don't engage in the battle. Offer a choice of *where* to settle down – bed, couch, etc. Or suggest that he *not* sleep; say it is okay just to rest his bones. If there is nothing to be gained from resisting you, he may give up the fight.

Alec wakes repeatedly during the night and just doesn't seem to need much sleep. I wonder if he would sleep better at night if I cut out his nap time?

This logic usually backfires. It is very easy for a child to become overly tired. Instead of making him sleepy, eliminating naptime will probably make him irritable and unable to settle down or sleep peacefully during the night.

Summary We have looked at common trouble spots that can disrupt a child's sleep. These trouble spots can be development-related (separation anxiety, nightmares, or sleep terrors), caused by a child's daily schedule (mealtimes or body rhythms), or simply be related to a child's personality and temperament (night owls and early risers).

Some issues show themselves during the day. A child may have a combination of difficulties or just one. If following the suggestions in this chapter don't bring changes, a more comprehensive process might be useful. Chapter 4 outlines four basic approaches and how each might be implemented.

Suggested Readings *Nightmare Help – for children, from children* by Anne Sayre Wiseman. Ten Speed Press, Berkeley, CA, 1989. UK distributor: Airlift Book Company, 26–28 Eden Grove, London N7 8EF.

Your Child's Dreams by Patricia Garfield, Ph.D. Ballantine, New York, 1984. UK distributor: Tiptree Book Services, Tiptree, Colchester CO5 0SR.

Growing Pains: Helping Children Deal with Everyday Problems through Reading by Maureen Cuddigan and Mary Beth Hanson. American Library Assoc., Chicago, 1988. UK distributor: International Book Distributors, Hemel Hempstead HP2 4RG.

Chapter 4 FOUR BASIC APPROACHES

When a *major* change is required, there are four basic approaches to solving family sleep problems. Each is described and summarized from a proponent's point of view. Some of the advantages and disadvantages are outlined. 'Points to Ponder' offers additional things to consider as you decide which approach best fits your family situation.

The Family Bed Approach

The custom of the mother, father, and young child sleeping together at night has been termed 'The Family Bed'. The basic belief is that babies desire and need to be closer to those who love them.

Philosophy   The basic idea of the Family Bed approach is that the whole family unit will work best if the needs of all members, including the children, are met. Taking cues from each other, the decision about the sleeping arrangements becomes a parenting decision based on how the family can best function – not on preconceived ideas about how families *should* sleep.

Often proposed by La Leche League, this method works easily with breast-feeding children. Another proponent, William Sears, a paediatrician and a father, sees the Family Bed as an integral part of parenting.

He interviewed over 5,000 parents about their experiences – what worked and what didn't – concerning sleep habits, problems, and solutions. In his book, *Night-time Parenting*, he describes the Family Bed more as an 'attitude' than a method. It fits a whole style of parenting called 'attachment parenting' where the members of the father-mother-child unit function together to understand and meet the baby's needs.

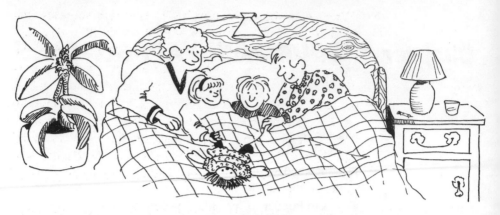

The Family Bed

Babies' needs do not stop at night, nor does parenting. Sears' goal is to help families achieve 'sleep harmony' so that the night-time experience becomes as valuable as the daytime experience. He recommends that parents welcome baby into their bed from birth to prevent potential sleep problems. Sleeping close to mum and getting needs met quickly helps babies organize their sleep patterns. After a year or so, their sleep patterns are more established. From one to three years, when children are awakened by other things, parents are reassuringly nearby.

Rob cried twenty-four hours a day for the first four months of his life. I can't remember it now without shuddering. The only time any of us got any sleep was when I was propped up on the bed with him lying across my stomach.

'High-need children' put special requirements on parents. They don't want to be put down; they cry inconsolably, have irregular patterns and rhythms, are extremely active, or are easily frustrated. Sleep problems are common. Attachment parenting helps parents meet those needs with the least amount of separation and stimulation for the child – and with the least physical and emotional drain on parents who are continually challenged.

The most common question about the Family Bed is

'When will she leave our bed?' Dr Sears suggests that *when* is not as important as *how*. As with other developmental issues, there is a wide variance between children. Parents' expectations or desires do not always dictate how the child develops. Wanting your child to walk on her birthday will not help if she is not ready. Similarly, she will reach the stage of independent sleeping when she is ready.

In his personal and professional experience, he has found that most children who have been part of the Family Bed since infancy leave voluntarily around their second or third year.

Following the guide of attachment parenting, a child will leave when her need has been satisfied. Sometimes there is a gradual weaning. She may sleep for a while in a sleeping bag on the floor of the parents' room, or she may sleep some nights in her own bed and some with parents or siblings. She may return periodically during times of stress.

Another common concern is the parents' need for privacy and to maintain a comfortable sex life. Using creativity in finding other times and places for lovemaking is one option. Moving a sleeping child to another room temporarily is another.

Parents' attitudes again come into play: if they see a child as an intrusion, this issue can cause conflict; if they view a strong parental bond as an equally important part of parenting, then they will find a way.

How to Proceed The arrangement is determined by the family's needs and lifestyle. It can range from taking baby into the parents' bed temporarily while he is being nursed and settled, to the building of a special bed that accommodates all family members for sleep. There are other possibilities in the middle of that range, such as simply welcoming children into the parents' bed during the night as the need arises, or setting up a mattress on the floor in their room.

One family's success. *Lexie was a frequent feeder, so I brought her to our bed to nurse while I dozed. We put her in her own room when she was about four months, but it* *seemed wrong to both of us. We decided she would stay with us until it caused problems, but she ended up staying there, comfortably for all of us, until she requested a 'big girl bed' at about age three.*

I guess the 'problems' all found solutions. We worried when she learned to crawl, but solved it by moving the bed against the wall. We had some mishaps during toilet training when she took off her nappies at night, but plastic sheets did the trick. We visited the guest room when we needed some 'privacy' – which made it more exciting! She still comes to us occasionally, and we welcome her without hardly waking up.

Pros & Cons

Advantages of the Family Bed Approach:

- Easy to feed upon demand.
- Less disruption of Mother and Father's sleep because they are able to respond without leaving the bed or waking fully.
- Increases amount of physical contact for baby.
- Decreases fear of falling asleep and dropping baby while nursing.
- Often increases amount of time Father spends near baby.
- Can coax early risers back to sleep.
- May increase bonding and development of intimacy.
- May increase closeness between siblings.
- May be the easiest way to meet extraordinary demands of high-need children.

Disadvantages of the Family Bed Approach:

- Decrease in parents' time alone.
- Movement or noise of some children can disrupt parents and vice versa.
- Hard for some women to find a comfortable sleeping/ nursing position.
- When used to sleeping with company, some children have difficulty napping or retiring alone if parents are otherwise engaged.
- Difficult for anyone other than parents to carry out;

therefore, it may be difficult to use a sitter or to be separated from children if necessary or desired.

- May be difficult to move into sleeping alone if this is the ultimate goal.

Points to Ponder

Whether an issue is seen as an advantage or a disadvantage can best be answered by individual families depending on their own values. Dr Sears points out that the Family Bed is not for everyone.

Tine Thevenin, in her book *The Family Bed*, discusses the difference between a need and a habit. She states:

The wants of a well-adjusted human being are his needs. It is when his needs are not fulfilled that his wants become excessive in the attempt to fulfil suppressed needs.[1]

This is probably the key philosophy that differentiates the Family Bed from other options. Assess your family values and lifestyle, your child's needs and temperament, and your own needs and temperament when you make your decision.

Cultural pressure is strong on both sides. Exercise 4.1 looks at ways to deal with criticism if you decide to use or adapt this approach. Parents who choose not to use this approach may feel guilty; sometimes a description of the Family Bed is so attractive that parents long for those good feelings. They wonder if they are not 'being there' emotionally for their child if they are not next to her physically. Once you've made a decision on a sleep plan for your family, spend your energy on implementing it instead of questioning your choice. No one knows your child, or yourselves, as well as you do – the decision is up to you. *Your* way is okay as long as it fits your family's needs.

Different preferences may exist between partners. It is common in families for one partner to be an advocate and the other an opponent to having children in the parental bed. The conflict that this creates often outweighs the advantages. If this is the case in your family, it is probably best to try a modified version or even one of the other possibilities. Special times can be set aside for children to spend in Mum and Dad's bed – weekend mornings, a special place to talk over private concerns, etc.

Remember, this is not an all-or-nothing proposition. Variations of the Family Bed are usually used by families at one time or another. As with other approaches, this can be viewed as a continuum – an approach that works with some families and at some times. It need not be a static solution, but part of an evolving process to be re-evaluated from time to time.

If you must face someone who is constantly critical, a support group like the La Leche League would lend some balance. Reading the books mentioned at the end of this chapter will help answer other questions. Generally, the more experience and success you build, the less impact criticism will have.

EXERCISE 4.1: Dealing With Others

Although shared sleeping is common in many cultures, it is no longer common in our society. The biggest challenge for parents who choose this approach is facing criticism from other people. Think about the ways you might respond to the following typical comments:

Aren't you afraid you will roll over and suffocate her?

I'd never let my child come between me and my husband – certainly not in bed!

You will never get him out of your bed. He will become too dependent on you.

How do you get any sleep?

The more comfortable you become with your position, the less you will feel the need to defend it. Talking with other parents who are experienced advocates is a good way to become comfortable. These attitudes might be helpful for you:

- Avoid being defensive. You'll never talk anyone into trying it, and convincing them isn't your goal anyway.
- It's your life and your decision. Sleep habits aren't generally something people discuss.
- Smile smugly – as if you have a secret the rest of the world is missing out on.
- Remember that Dr Sears' experience has shown The Family Bed brings the quickest results in decreasing crying (not associated with separation issues).

The Cry It Out Approach

The basic belief of this approach is that children can and will learn appropriate sleep patterns when inappropriate tendencies are not reinforced by attention from parents. The child cries in protest while he is learning to fall asleep on his own.

Philosophy   There are two beliefs that support the Cry It Out approach. First, unwanted behaviour that is ignored will die out; and second, a reasonable amount of crying does not hurt a child.

Dr Burton White, author of *The First Three Years of Life*, is one of the proponents of this method. After working with hundreds of families using this method, he has found no observable disturbances in the child's emotional well-being. He feels that this approach fits consistently with a good understanding of early childhood development. Dr White assures us that, for a healthy, normal child, this method will be successful if carried out for seven to ten days.

Dr Marc Weissbluth, Director of the Sleep Disorders Center in Chicago, feels parents interfere with natural and

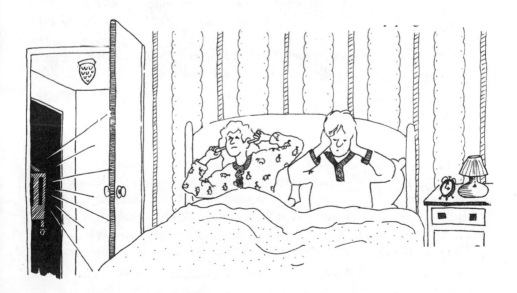

important learning of the four-to-twelve-month-old child by being actively involved in the going-to-sleep process. He states (and quotes several other professionals) that not responding to a 'protest cry' will *not* produce insecurity when parents are normally nurturing during the day. On the contrary, the absence of healthy sleep habits is more harmful.

How to Proceed

After a bedtime ritual, the parent leaves the room and allows the child to cry until he falls asleep – no maximum amount of time for crying is set. The same approach is used each time the child is put to bed or wakes. The parent responds promptly to the first cry to make sure there is nothing 'wrong' – such as illness. The prediction is that with each incident the length of crying will decrease and the child will learn to put himself to sleep until the night wakings disappear altogether.

One family's success. *When ten-month-old Christina woke twice a night, each time her father walked her until she fell asleep. Christina had learned that her father would be there to ease her back to sleep. To change this, her parents decided she needed to cry it out. Because dad's presence was the most comforting, dad began the programme.*

The first night, dad walked her until she was sleepy, then laid her in her cot awake. Understandably upset, she cried for almost an hour. She woke only once that night. Dad checked briefly on her, laid her down, and left the room. Again, she cried for close to an hour.

The second night she cried for 45 minutes at bedtime and 40 minutes during the night. Although it was hard for her parents, her father told himself that he often had spent up to that much time awake walking her.

The third night, she cried for 20 minutes at bedtime and only briefly during the night. Because she was not crying hard and they were assured of her health and safety, they chose not to check on her at all. The fourth night she cried softly for 10 minutes and did not wake at night. The fifth night, she went down with only a whimper and slept until morning.

Pros & Cons

Advantages of the Cry It Out Approach:

- Comparatively quick results – usually within a week, sometimes after only three days.
- The least complicated plan; has little room for additional decisions while implementing it.
- The least amount of parental involvement; it relies on the child's ability to deal with the problem in his own way.
- History shows this has worked with many families.

Disadvantages of the Cry It Out Approach:

- Can be very difficult for parents with a low tolerance for crying. There is a tendency to abandon the plan in the middle before any progress is made.
- Works best with child still in a cot. Room modifications must be made for a child who gets out of bed.
- Can be very noisy.
- Parents tend to have fears/fantasies about what is going on in the child's room. The temptation to check or comfort sabotages the plan.
- Parents sometimes feel guilt – as if they are abandoning their child.

Points to Ponder

The experience of respected experts should alleviate the common concern that your child will feel abandoned or develop deep-seated emotional problems by crying himself to sleep. The difficulty may begin when, no matter how logical or 'right' parents *know* this method is, there are some people who simply cannot do it. Sometimes parents try it one night and decide that the child can outlast them – which may, indeed, be true.

Frequently partners have very different temperaments and tolerance for crying. At no time will differences seem so monumental than in the middle of the night. Better to talk about religion or politics than to work on your plan in the middle of a crying session. It is crucial to success that it be discussed and discussed again before implementing it. It will not work in a two-partner family if only one partner is invested in it. See Exercise 4.2 for ideas

EXERCISE 4.2: Preparation For Cry It Out

The biggest challenge facing parents who choose to let their child cry it out is dealing with their own emotional distress. This approach fails when parents feel they can't follow through. Having supports ready ahead of time is the best way to make it work.

Here are four areas to think about before you begin. Check the items that you might find helpful. Add your own ideas.

1. Prepare The Environment To Muffle Noise.

There are ways to alter the setting to make the crying more tolerable.

____ Tuck blankets around the door   ____ Hang blankets around windows
____ Turn on the radio for 'white noise'   ____ Put a rug or blanket on the floor
                                                  of the child's room

2. Prepare People Involved.

____ Talk to your neighbours ahead of time   ____ Move siblings to another room

3. Prepare Yourself.

Parents can choose to pamper, distract, or purposefully make themselves miserable when carrying out this plan.

____ Turn on the TV   ____ Visualize or wish your child into
____ Start reading a new book   sleep
____ Work on a project   ____ Pace the floor, tear paper
____ Give yourself permission to eat,   ____ Talk on the telephone
      smoke, bite your nails, etc.   ____ Arrange for a supportive friend
____ Cry   to visit
____ Go outside   ____ Stare at the clock and wait for
                                                  the crying to diminish

4. Prepare Your Partner.

In a two-partner family, this approach works best if both parents are committed to it. However, it is not often that simple. Parents have different ways of handling stress and different levels of tolerance for crying.

____ Discuss ahead of time your   ____ Agree that one person will
      individual ways of coping with   handle it. Perhaps arrange for
      stress   the other person not to be at
____ Realize that this will be a temporary   home
      situation – irrational behaviour will   ____ Arrange for some 'special time'
      not be held against each other   together or with your child
      later   during the day
____ Leave each other alone   ____ Choose a weekend or a time
____ Work out in advance each partner's   when you don't need as much
      role in the plan   sleep, or when it might be easier
____ Hold each other   for both parents to be involved

on how to prepare your child, yourself, and your family.

If you are sure that your child will hate you in the morning, take special note of how quickly the grin returns when she wakes up. In the long run, children welcome the limits parents put on their world. The message you are giving is:

I know you can do it. I support you, but I will not hinder you by doing the things for you that you can best do on your own.

The Teaching in Small Steps Approach

The basis of this method is the belief that a child learns best when new expectations are presented gradually. Since he is accustomed to a certain sleep pattern, he need not be cut off completely, but can learn by taking steps toward the goal. His parents become less and less involved in the process while the child learns to depend on his own resources.

This method has unlimited variations and can be used for many different problems. First, we will look at its application to teach a child to get to, and back to, sleep on his own. Variations will be discussed later.

Philosophy The basic belief of the Small Steps approach is that given time and encouragement, a child will develop his own resources and style for getting to sleep.

This method works well for the child who is accustomed to his parent's help or presence to get to sleep. The parent puts the child in his own bed and then, as he cries, progressively lengthens the intervals between checking on him until he falls asleep.

Visits from the parent come just often enough to show that they are 'still out there'. The time between visits becomes longer and longer so that the visits themselves do not become reinforcing. Both child and parent are gradually learning to tolerate longer and longer separations.

The parent's role is to continue to provide encouragement, without 'helping' the child in the process of going to sleep itself. The child will understandably be unhappy, but he will not feel deserted. There may be some crying, but the idea is not that he cries himself to the point of exhaustion. He develops his own way to get to sleep. Some children 'nest' amongst the blankets. Others cuddle a special toy or suck their thumbs. Others simply lie down and go to sleep.

Dr Richard Ferber, as a proponent of this method, believes that a child's sleep associations need not include his parents – that 'help' most often becomes a hindrance. He has found this approach to be highly successful with numerous families. Young babies show improvement within a few days or certainly within a week. Older children may take slightly longer, but are just as successful.

Another proponent is Penelope Leach, author of *Your Baby and Child: From Birth to Five.* She recommends simply checking in with the child at steady five-minute intervals.

Dr T. Berry Brazelton recommends that, after going to a child several times, a parent simply call out reassuringly to the child without going into his room. He stresses that teaching attachment to a 'lovey' is an important part of the teaching process.

How to Proceed Parents begin by deciding just how much crying they think they can tolerate – that becomes the maximum for the first night. The minimum is usually set at 5 minutes or less if need be. They set up an environment that is safe, comfortable, and equipped with whatever they feel will help their child to settle himself independently. Using a brief, calming night-time ritual, a parent puts the child down in his own bed. The child is allowed to fuss for the minimum time. Then a parent goes to the child and, taking only one or two minutes, gives a word or pat of firm, confident reassurance and leaves the room.

Using the progressive method, the intervals increase in 5 minute increments as follows:

Day one: 5, 10, 15, 15, 15 as needed.
Day two: 10, 15, 20, 20, 20 as needed.
Day three: 15, 20, 25, 25, 25 as needed.

At bedtime or in the middle of the night, the programme continues until the child falls asleep, or is no longer crying vigorously. Notice that, on the following night, the beginning interval is longer as parents, too, are building their own tolerance. The child learns that the visits are less frequent.

At naptime, the programme continues for an hour. If the child has not gone to sleep by that time, you get him out of bed. So that your programme later that evening will not suffer, follow the hour rule no matter how long his usual naptime is.

In two-parent families, parents can take turns responding to the child (each night or alternate nights). This takes some pressure off one parent, and ensures that one parent doesn't become part of the sleep associations.

The checking times are soothing, but need not end the crying. The parent should *not* be present when the child goes to sleep.

One family's success. *Eighteen-month-old Bruce was accustomed to being rocked to sleep. His dad continued to use rocking as part of the bedtime ritual, but laid him down to sleep when he was drowsy and still awake. Dad left the room and Bruce cried for 5 minutes. Dad returned, handed him his stuffed bear with some words of encouragement, and left for 10 minutes. His maximum wait time that night was 20 minutes – it took three 20-minute sessions.*

The next night, Dad began checking after 10 minutes and worked up to one, 25-minute session. Bruce was whimpering instead of screaming, so Dad did not go back in.

The third night, Bruce cried for the first 15 minutes. After Dad checked on him, he began sobbing loudly – but settled down after a few minutes. Dad did not need to return.

The fourth and final night, Bruce called out when he was first put down, but went quickly to sleep.

Variations of the basic plan are endless. They can be devised according to the situation and temperaments of all people involved. They can take as long as you, and the child, have patience.

Child who has been 'helped' to sleep. If your child has become accustomed to being fed, rocked, or otherwise helped to sleep, you may feel that simply putting him to bed wide awake is too extreme. It is not unreasonable for you to have difficulty with even five minutes of crying. You can begin with some preparatory steps.

For Andrew, my goal was to get him to sleep without nursing. Instead of tiptoeing to his room when he finished eating, I purposefully roused him. Then I laid him in his bed and patted his back until he was asleep. When I felt he was comfortable with the idea of sleeping lying down instead of in my arms, I gradually began leaving him sooner and sooner. We worked up to just laying him down, giving a brief pat, and leaving the room. It still works for him.

The ultimate goal is still the same: the child will learn to get to sleep by himself. The short-term goal is to accustom him to going to sleep in his bed. After laying him down, offer the minimum interaction that will make him or yourself comfortable. As nights proceed, lessen your involvement until it is minimal or virtually non-existent.

Child who needs you to sleep with her. An older child who is used to your being with her while she goes to sleep can be weaned from your presence. If she is old enough, explain what you will be working on. Make it sound positive

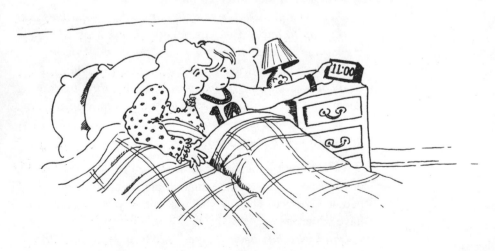

'He's awake again?'

– something you will be working on together, slowly. Build on positive feelings – you can do it! Try not to communicate rejection, but rather confidence in her ability.

Begin by sitting on a chair next to her bed. As nights pass, move the chair farther away from her bed and closer to the door. Depending on the child, you might sit on the chair outside her room for a while. She ultimately learns that she can go to sleep in her own room without you.

If she demands that you lie down with her or if she gets out of bed, explain that you will stay in the room sitting on the chair or you will leave the room. The choice is hers. Keeping you there – even if you are not in her bed – is usually more attractive to her than having you leave.

Child with unusual sleep cycle. Changing an internal clock needs to be done slowly to allow the body to catch up. This method is described in Chapter 3.

Child who learned unwanted habits after an illness. A gradual process is appropriate when you are concerned about health – or any other time when your sympathy might keep you from making changes.

Pros & Cons   **Advantages of the Small Steps Approach:**

- Appropriate after a child reaches about five or six months.
- Meets the emotional needs of parents and child; it doesn't feel extreme and parents seldom feel that they are deserting the child.
- Because parents can check in on the child, their fears and fantasies about what is going on are relieved.
- Particularly suited to children going through separation issues.
- Can be tailored to the individuals and situations involved.
- Someone other than parents will be able to put the child to sleep.

Disadvantages of the Small Steps Approach:

- Depending on the particular plan, it may take longer than other methods.

- Some children are upset rather than comforted by the sight of their parents.
- Some parents weaken at the sight of their child in distress and may abandon the plan.
- Parents need to tolerate a certain amount of crying.
- This approach is more parent-centred than child-centred.

EXERCISE 4.3: Determining The Small Steps

For practice in teaching small steps toward a 'sleeping' goal, outline several steps you might use in these situations. There are many possibilities – none right or wrong. Some suggestions are given.

Current state: **Ultimate Goal:**

Rocking to sleep . . . . Laying down to sleep

_____

_____

_____

_____

Riding in car until asleep . . . . Laying down to sleep in bed

_____

_____

_____

_____

Possible plans:

Rocking: Plan A – Rock until child is drowsy; rock child briefly; sit still in rocking chair with child for a minute; remove rocker from sight. *Plan B* – Stop rocking at morning nap; stop rocking at afternoon nap.

Riding: Plan A – Ride in car to be sure he is sleepy; bring child in the house and rock him to sleep; rock to sleep without car. *Plan B* – Jiggle his bed until he's asleep; jiggle until he's drowsy.

Points to   Making changes in small steps offers an alternative for those
Ponder   parents who, for whatever reason, do not feel comfortable
either letting their child cry it out or taking him into their
own bed. It gives the parents flexibility to personalize their
plan, to take it as slowly or quickly as they want.

Parents who might have wanted to, but felt they couldn't
tolerate *any* crying, are able to successfully follow through
because their expectations for themselves are broken down
into small steps. Each step feels like a big accomplishment.
Parents can even institute a reward system for each small
step achieved.

**Parents take an active part in finding a solution and
carrying it out.** They lose their sense of helplessness. The
role of teacher or guide is one that usually fits parents well.
Although this plan seems highly structured, many parents
already instinctively check on and reassure their fussing
child. Discovering that this is an actual 'method' relieves the
guilt that some parents express about feeling the need to
check in. The progressive component of lengthening times
before checking adds to the learning process for the child.

The Living With It Approach

Philosophy   There are many reasons why a family might choose to
simply live with the current sleep situation and make the
best of things the way they are.

- Perhaps you are waiting for life circumstances to change
  – you will be moving soon, a new baby is expected or has
  just arrived, you will be returning to work, or changing
  day care. If you know that your life will soon be in
  upheaval, you may as well wait until routine is re-estab-
  lished. Some children tend to be upset by change and
  show their feelings through sleep disturbances.
- Parents may feel that their child's sleep patterns are tied
  too closely to his personality or individual circumstances
  to warrant asking for a change. They feel it is easier for
  them to learn to live with the situation than it would be to
  expect the child to make changes. This child may be

EXERCISE 4.4: Which Method Will Work Best For Us?

Each approach has different characteristics. Part of being successful is choosing the plan that best fits each family's needs and beliefs. To help you distinguish the differences and to find the best 'match' for you, read the following statements and choose the approach or approaches that might be the most suitable.
Key: (F= Family Bed, C= Cry It Out, T= Teaching in Small Steps.)

_____ 1. I can't stand to hear my child cry.

_____ 2. I need my privacy.

_____ 3. We travel a lot without our children.

_____ 4. I am a light sleeper, easily disturbed.

_____ 5. We go out in the evening and use a babysitter to put the kids to bed.

_____ 6. I feel that a little crying is okay, maybe even necessary.

_____ 7. I need a full night of uninterrupted sleep to be at my best during the day.

_____ 8. I enjoy sleeping with my children near me.

_____ 9. I feel it is important to respond to each cry.

_____ 10. I worry if my children are far from me.

_____ 11. We live in close quarters and I am concerned about waking the rest of the family, or the neighbours.

_____ 12. Privacy with my partner in our bed is a priority for me.

_____ 13. I don't spend as much time with my child during the day as I would like.

_____ 14. I want a solution as quickly as possible.

_____ 15. I could handle a few nights of crying if it means that sleep will follow.

Answers to this exercise are subjective; since they are opinions there are no right or wrong answers. Compare your responses with these guidelines: 1. F,T; 2. C,T; 3. T; 4. C,T; 5. C,T; 6. C,T; 7. C,T (Parents who get their best sleep *with* children will also mark this F); 8. F; 9. F,T; 10. F; 11. F,T; 12. C,T; 13. F; 14. C,F; 15. C,T.

described as 'high need' or emotionally fragile. He may have a history of serious illness or be continually illness-prone. The parents are reluctant to ask him to be more independent at this time.

- Sometimes the parents' own temperaments or values convince them that it would be better to leave the situation the way it is. Perhaps none of the choices feels 'right'. They may have tried several things already and nothing has worked.
- The 'readiness factor' isn't right yet. The parents don't

plan to wait forever and don't plan to *never* make changes, but they know that, for now, they are not ready. Sometimes these parents are waiting for things to get better on their own.

How to Proceed

You've decided to live with it. Don't fight it. Accept it as a conscious decision and try not to feel guilty. Begin making adjustments in your life that will make it easier to cope.

The first step is to chart current sleep patterns for about three days. This will help you see the situation clearly and perhaps identify places for minor changes.

Develop some support systems. When you feel that your nights are a battle or are constantly interrupted, the natural reaction is to feel burdened, abused, or angry. Find some ways to get your own needs met during the day.

Work out a system to handle the night-time disturbances. There are various ways to divide or share night-time duty with your partner. Father might take responsibility for the first half of the night and mother the second half – leaving one of you relatively undisturbed for at least part of the night. Or each of you might be on duty every other night. Decide who gets to sleep in and who gets morning duty on which days. Watch your own anger – especially blaming each other. Make sure both of you are committed to living with it. Set a time in the future to reassess the situation.

One family's success. *Hannah was seriously asthmatic and could barely be left alone at night. John and I traded half nights – he took the first shift, I took the second. I took the weekends so he could catch up on sleep. We hired a babysitter for me to take an afternoon nap three times a week. We cut out as many morning activities as possible – John even arranged to go into work an hour and a half later. We also made a special effort to spend more time alone together to support each other. It was the only way we could have lived through the first couple of years.*

Pros & Cons

Advantages of the Living With It Approach:

- Gives parents time to re-think situation.
- Allows time for situation to improve on its own.

- The conscious decision decreases parents' feeling of powerlessness.
- Takes pressure off parents to 'do something' or 'fix it'.
- Decreases guilt – focuses on problem, not parents.

Disadvantages of the Living With It Approach:

- Passage of time doesn't always solve the problem.
- May only put off the inevitable.
- This approach is easily confused with 'doing nothing' – which increases risk of failure.
- Can be difficult to keep your feelings in check for too long or when sleep deprivation continues.

Points to Ponder

There are those times when learning to live with it is the best solution – sometimes temporarily, sometimes longer. Look closely at your motives and reasoning. Weigh the effects on your life, on your child, and on the whole family. Continue to re-evaluate the situation periodically since children change constantly in their sleep needs and in their ability to handle new situations and new challenges.

There is an expression, 'Not to decide is to decide.' Recognize that, even temporarily, you have chosen not to take steps for changes, and that is okay. Then make the adjustments that can make life more bearable.

Summary

Each of the approaches is 'tried and true'. Choose the one that works for you. You may already think one approach is bizarre, while another strikes you as possible. One approach may work well with one child, but not at all with his sibling. Continue to re-evaluate your choices as your child grows older. A different approach may be more workable later, if there are still problems.

The next step is to take the basic information and develop your own personalized approach, to fit your child's sleep problem. Chapter 5 will lead you through that process.

Suggested Reading

Dr Spock on Parenting by Benjamin Spock, M.D. Michael Joseph, London, 1989.

The Family Bed: An Age-old Concept in Childrearing by Tine Thevenin. Avery Publishing Group, Wayne, NJ, 1987. UK distributor: Worldwide Media Service, Partridge Green, W. Sussex RH13 8LD.

The First Three Years of Life by Burton L. White, M.D. W. H. Allen, London, 1978.

Healthy Sleep Habits, Happy Child by Marc Weissbluth, M.D. Fawcett Columbine, New York, 1987. UK distributor: Tiptree Book Services, Tiptree, Colchester CO5 0SR.

Nighttime Parenting: How to Get Your Baby and Child to Sleep by William Sears, M.D. New American Library, New York, 1987. UK distributor: Penguin Books, Harmondsworth UB7 0DA.

To Listen to a Child by T. Berry Brazelton, M.D. Addison-Wesley, Reading, MA, 1984. UK distributor: Southport Book Distributors, Southport PR9 9YF.

Your Baby and Child: From Birth to Age Five by Penelope Leach. Michael Joseph, London, 1977.

The Womanly Art of Breastfeeding by La Leche League International. New American Library, New York, 1987. UK distributor: Penguin Books, Harmondsworth UB7 0DA.

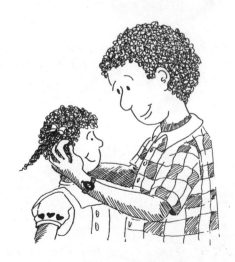

'Let's work on it together.'

Chapter 5 PLAN FOR SUCCESS

This chapter takes you through the problem-solving steps. The process includes gathering data, defining the problem, looking at alternatives, deciding on a plan, putting the plan into action, reviewing the situation and revising the plan, and congratulating yourself. Read them through so you can think about the whole process before you begin to make changes.

Develop a Sleep Plan

A 'sleep plan' is a strategy that parents develop to tackle the sleep problems in their family. It is based on current information about sleep. It looks at the specific situation: type of problem, age of child, and family circumstances. It takes into account the family goals and values.

An individualized plan has a much greater chance for success than simply jumping in and trying anything. What you try out of desperation may not bring the long-term solution you desire. What worked for your nephew may not work for your son.

STEP 1: Gather Date

To solve your sleep problem you need to collect both historical and current information.

Start at the beginning. Look at your child's sleep history. In Exercise 2.4 you charted your child's patterns from birth. Go back to that chart and summarize the patterns. For example:

Nicholas slept through the night when he was young. The problem (waking up screaming) began about a year ago.

Look at what is happening now. It is tempting to jump into working on the problem without figuring out where you are now. But taking this step is crucial. You will form a baseline to make comparisons and note changes. Some-

83

times just writing it down makes the problem seem more manageable.

Using Exercise 5.1, record your child's current sleep patterns. Take an average day, or (much better) take three days and note his day and night schedule. Note times of getting to sleep and waking. If he is young or if you suspect feeding may be part of the problem, include times of feeding. Include any other information that you feel might be pertinent. There's no need to be elaborate. It is important to make this chart even if it is only jotting down notes on a pad by your bed.

Expectations. *Compare your child's current patterns with what is considered 'average' in order to set realistic expectations. Check the Average Sleep Needs chart in Chapter 2 to review what is normal at different ages.*

STEP 2: Define the Problem

Go back to your chart and put a star by those times of the day or night that bother you. The problem might be the timing, attitude, or environment.

Define the problem as specifically as you can. Using the information you have gathered so far, decide what is *not* acceptable to you about your child's sleep habits. Make a list of problems in all areas. Describe specifics exactly. For example: *She does not go to sleep without a fight.* **Or,** *He wakes too often at night. That is, he wakes two times a night. At his age I don't think he should wake at all.*

Return to *Types of Sleep Problems* described in Chapter 1. Decide which of them fit the problems you listed (there may be more than one). For example: *She does not go to sleep without a fight = difficulty getting to sleep alone.* Or, *He wakes too often at night = frequent waking.*

Set Goals. Knowing what is unacceptable, decide what you would like to work towards. Relate directly back to the problem as you defined it. Be as specific as possible. For example: *Bedtime will go smoothly, without hassles.* Or, *No night waking.*

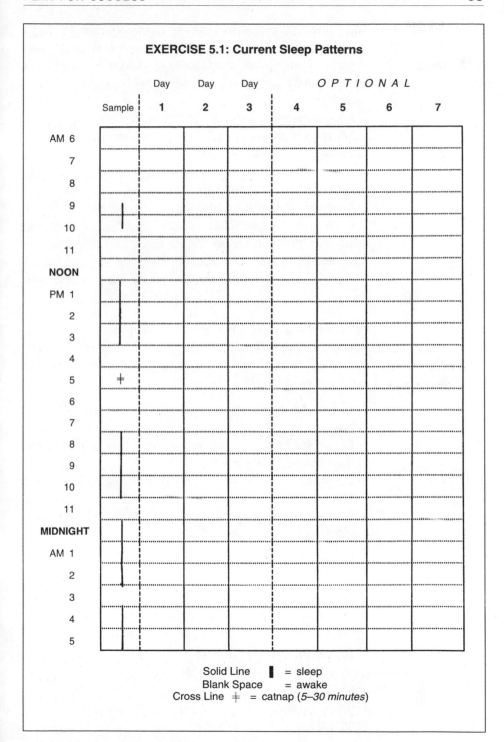

EXERCISE 5.1: Current Sleep Patterns

Solid Line █ = sleep
Blank Space = awake
Cross Line ╪ = catnap (*5–30 minutes*)

STEP 3:
Look at
Alternatives

Sometimes the goal seems too big or overwhelming. If you break it down into steps, it becomes more manageable and realistic. Think about what skills your child needs to learn in order to reach that goal. One step builds on another. For example:

Long-term goal: He will sleep through the night.

Short-term steps: First, he needs to learn to get back to sleep on his own after he wakes during the night. Second, he needs to learn to get to sleep on his own at sleep times – in his own bed and without parents present.

Your thinking will be like that of any teacher. To teach your child to play basketball you could put him in a gym and throw him the ball. Or you might teach him to dribble, to pass, and to shoot. Your teaching style will depend on the skills you think are important, his natural abilities, and your values.

Small changes can make a big difference. The suggestions in Chapter 3 may set the stage (or, in some cases, eliminate the need) for a major approach. Here are some possibilities to check:

- Check daytime routine (irregular, no naps, too many naps).
- Check feeding habits (lengthen time between feedings, decrease night feedings).
- Encourage attachment to 'lovey' (decrease fears, ease separation).
- Check bedtime routine (lengthen, shorten, make more independent).
- Check environment (noise, light, temperature, scary).
- Make new sleep associations (parent less involved, try 'lovey').
- Check for developmental disequilibrium (be patient, teach coping skills).

Remember, make only one change at a time. Try the change for one week. If you can't continue that long, go at least four days. Change takes a while – especially if your child is tenacious! Avoid the common tendency to try it once and say, 'That didn't work.'

**STEP 4:
Decide on a
Plan**

You will want a more major approach when the suggestions from Chapter 3 have not worked, or when you feel the problem is more pervasive or tenacious.

Choose one of the four basic approaches summarized in Chapter 4. You will want to consider: the type of problem, your child's age and temperament, and your own values and temperament. Exercise 4.4 will help you clarify your goals for your family.

Set the scene.   You can 'stack the deck for success' by setting the scene carefully before you begin.

Physical setting: Make the sleep setting safe and comfortable. If you do it in advance, you won't question it later – or feel guilty that you haven't done enough. For example, you needn't worry if he has lost his covers if he is dressed in a blanket sleeper.

If noise is a problem, arrange makeshift sound barriers. Explain your plan and intentions to your neighbours so that you will not be swayed by a complaint or question.

Family members: Enlist cooperation from your partner and children. Establish tasks so everyone knows what to do.

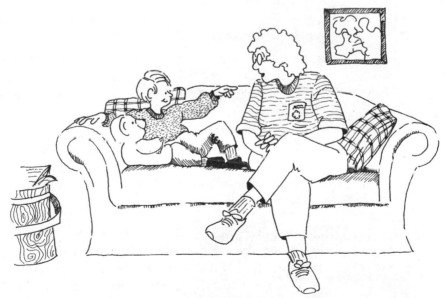

Prepare your child for the night-time changes.

EXERCISE 5.2: Plan For Success

Use the seven steps below to think about your family's sleep problem and develop a plan.

1. Gather Data.
   What have your child's sleep habits been like?

   What sleep habits do you expect of your child?

2. Define the Problem (be specific).
   Short description of the problem.

   Goal for your child or family.

     Short-term.

     Long-term.

3. List alternatives. (As many as you can: simple or complex, possible or improbable.)

4. Choose a plan & plan for success.
   I will begin by:
   If needed, I will:

   To improve our chance of success I will need to:
     [ ] Arrange the physical setting.
     [ ] Involve family members.
     [ ] Check timing (plan when to start).
     [ ] Arrange for personal support.
     [ ] Prepare the child.

5. Put plan in action.
   We will begin:

6. Evaluate your process & revise the plan.
   Date planned (Continue revising as necessary.)

7. Congratulate yourself and your child!!

Explain to siblings what is going on and why. Make temporary arrangements, if necessary, for children who share a bedroom.

Timing: Start on a weekend or another time when you won't feel pressure to get enough sleep. Be sure *you* will be there until the initial learning is done – don't ask a sitter to participate in the plan.

Support systems: Call friends, alert neighbours, bake cookies. Make ready whatever is comforting to you.

Prepare the child: Explain to your child what you are going to do and why. If the child is old enough, talk in gentle terms of doing it together and helping him learn so that he does not feel punished. Nothing will be gained by apologizing or talking in patronizing tones. Instead, talk with confidence so that he will be assured of his safety and your good wishes. Even if he is not old enough to completely understand, he will, at some level, know that something different, and not bad, will be happening. Plan for positive, nurturing daytime experiences for you and your partner to share with your child.

STEP 5: Put the Plan into Action

Putting your plan into action takes patience, persistence, and belief in your child and yourself.

Decide how long you will continue with the plan. A good rule of thumb is to give it a full week. Fight the temptation to try it once and give up; almost nothing works the first time. Your hope that the plan will work quickly doesn't give your child any credit for having determination! Parents who have a long list of things they have tried probably have not tried one thing for long enough. Set the date and begin.

Children change in different ways. Some children make logical, progressive changes. Each night gets easier than the last. Others will struggle from the beginning and continue to struggle until they make the change. Still other children begin relatively smoothly and then suddenly resist – which can raise doubts as to whether or not you are doing the right thing. This frequently happens on the third night. You, very understandably, will want to give up. However, if you can get through it, this is often the last push before the big change occurs.

STEP 6:
Evaluate the
Situation

Have you reached your goal? If so, pat yourself on the back. How does your child feel? Sometimes it is entirely appropriate to decide to change your plan. You can do so without feeling that you have failed or given up.

Sometimes there are things you just couldn't know until you started. Perhaps you gained new insights about yourself, your temperament, or expectations. Or you have new

---

EXERCISE 5.3: How Does My Plan Feel To Me?

Now that you are ready to start, take a minute to go through this checklist to make sure that your expectations are realistic and the environment is supportive. Check all the considerations that are true for you and your family.

_____ 1. **Child's age:** are your expectations appropriate for your child's age and developmental level?

_____ 2. **Child's temperament:** how do you think he will respond?

_____ 3. **Parents' temperament:** what is your tolerance for crying, noise, lack of sleep?

_____ 4. **Partners:** are both ready to support and carry out the plan? Or is there agreement to let one partner handle it?

_____ 5. **Siblings:** are they prepared for how the plan may affect parents, themselves, and the child?

_____ 6. **Living arrangement:** does it need any revision to ensure the plan's success?

_____ 7. **Lifestyle:** does the plan or the outcome fit the way you live and the things that are important to you?

_____ 8. **Time frame:** how desperate are you? Do you need resolution as soon as possible, or are you willing to make gradual changes that may take longer?

_____ 9. **Trouble shooting:** are you ready? What could possibly go awry, and how could you lessen the possibilities before you begin?

_____ 10. **Self-care:** are all of your own support systems ready to help you follow through?

information about your child, her needs, problem area, or temperament.

The timing might be wrong. The child or parent may have been ill. Upsetting life experiences might have occurred. Siblings might have interfered. You may not be committed to carrying it out. Were you talked into something you didn't agree with? Were you trying to prove something to yourself or someone else?

You may now know that your goals were not realistic and you want to re-evaluate them, perhaps even begin again. Perhaps you thought you needed to be (or could be) 'brave' or 'tough', but now feel you can't or don't want to. Maybe you thought you wanted to take it slowly, but you just got frustrated and took a big leap.

Revise your plan, if necessary. Don't give up! You have come too far. In fact, you are now further ahead – even though you may not feel that way. Give yourself credit for being flexible and resourceful enough to change your plan if it needs it.

Use the information you gained to make the changes, if necessary. Here are a few suggestions:

Timing: Something has come up – perhaps illness or a change of day care. When (be as specific as possible) will the conflicting issue be resolved?

Temperament: Would one of the other approaches be more suited to you or your child's temperament? Would things go more easily or smoothly (faster or slower) if you tried a different approach?

Review your expectations: Be sure you are working on what you *want* to be working on. For example, don't work on sleeping all night when you think she might still be hungry at 2:00 a.m.

Continue your programme. Unless timing was the issue, continue with your programme as soon as possible. If there is a very long break, it will be like beginning again. The child will be confused – and perhaps more stubborn. Or you might lose your momentum.

STEP 7:
Congratulate
Yourself

You did it! Take a minute to look at where you and your child came from – and where you are now. Pat yourselves on the back – your child included. It may not have been easy for any of you. Take special notice of changes you will begin to see in yourselves as parents as you get more sleep or have fewer battles. Notice changes in your child. If you expected him to feel angry or clingy, you will probably see other things – a more even temperament or a more predictable schedule. The benefits will soon compensate for the hard work you put into your plan.

A look to the future. When you have reached your goal, celebrate – and remain watchful. The recurrence of sleep problems is quite common. It is evidence of the fact that people don't grow on neat, charted paths, but in a series of up-and-down, back-and-forth steps. For some children with a history of sleep disturbance, the area of sleep is a 'weak spot'. Sleep becomes difficult at times when life is more demanding or exciting, or during new growth.

Don't panic. Give the situation some time before deciding that a new pattern is emerging. If things don't return to normal when the difficult time passes, a firm approach will get things back on track.

Return to the tactic that worked before – or something similar. The child will be reassured and can make use of past learning. You will also be comfortable and it will take less planning on your part. It is also not uncommon to take a firmer stance.

Be wary of doing *too much*. Have faith in your child. She will find it reassuring to know the ground rules haven't changed.

Summary

Remember, the problem-solving process involves gathering data, defining the problem, looking at alternatives, deciding on a plan, putting the plan into action, and reviewing and revising the plan. To make this process more concrete, the next chapter will illustrate how five different families might use these approaches with their children.

Chapter 6 PUT THEORY INTO PRACTICE

To bring these ideas closer to home, let's look at how three families proceeded. These families were not chosen because they are testimonials to the 'pure' methods outlined. Instead, they are examples of finding the 'process'. They demonstrate their own ways of working things through, and they show different methods, problems, and ages of children.

Teaching in Small Steps Approach

Christopher, age 26 months, is now a toddler. Because his frequent night waking has occurred since infancy, his mother will take a slower method to teach the independent sleep habits which he's never acquired.

Gather Data First we will look at the background of the problem, and then what the parents want to change.

History: Christopher was a 'newborn delight' who slept eight hours a night from the time he came home from the hospital. When he was about 9 months old, separation difficulties peaked and he demanded his mother's presence several times a night. She responded to him as needed. The waking became a pattern.

Current sleep patterns: He still wakes once or twice a night. His mother sits by his cot and pats him until he goes back to sleep. This takes from 30 minutes to one hour.

His mother is now a single parent to Christopher and his sister who share a room. When he wakes his sister, their mother must deal with both of them.

Expectations: For his age: 10 to 12 hours a night of uninterrupted sleep.

Define the Problem

Let's assess the problem areas:

- Frequent waking and difficulty falling asleep after waking.

Long-term goal: He will sleep all night or will be able to get himself back to sleep after waking.

Short-term goal: He will learn new sleep associations that do not involve his mother.

Look at Alternatives

Christopher's mother looks at both small scale alternatives and major change alternatives.

Small Scale Approaches: *Attachment to love objects* – Christopher has a favourite blanket. She begins teaching him to associate it with comfort and sleep by including it in bedtime rituals and special quiet times.

Major Change Approaches: Christopher's mother considers the Family Bed, Cry It Out, and Teaching in Small Steps approaches.

Decide on a Plan

Mother feels he is too old to begin Family Bed. She feels he is still too prone to separation issues to let him cry it out. She will teach new sleep habits using small steps.

Put the Plan into Action

Christopher's mother looks at preparing for the plan as well as implementing the plan itself.

Set the scene: She begins on a weekend so that Christopher's sister can spend the night away from home. Mother invites a friend to stay with her so she has some adult support while she puts the plan into action. She spends special time with Christopher during the day to reassure him that cuddling can continue – just not during the night.

Plan in action: Friday, Christopher wakes once at 4:00 a.m. Mother goes to him, gives him his blanket, lays him down with the reassuring words 'more night-night' and leaves the room – even though he hops up and cries. She uses the same tactic at increasing intervals: 5, 7, 10, and 15 minutes. Fifteen minutes is her maximum that night, but he continues to cry. After three 15-minute-sessions, he quiets to a whimper. She does not go in again and he falls asleep.

Saturday, he wakes three times. She begins checking after 7, 10, and 15 minutes to her maximum of 20. The first waking takes two 20-minute sessions. The second waking (beginning again at 7 minutes) also takes two 20-minute sessions. After the third waking, he falls asleep after the 10-minute check.

Sunday, he wakes once. She checks at 10, 15, 20, and 25 minutes and then he falls asleep. Monday he wakes once again. Not sure if she can continue much longer, she is surprised when he quiets down after the 10-minute check. She resists checking on him for half an hour. When she finds he is asleep, she is optimistic about the next night. On Tuesday, exhausted, she calls to him 'more night-night' and he settles down after a few minutes. This continues a couple of days until he stops waking her entirely.

Evaluate the Situation   Although it took intensive effort on her part, Mother feels the plan was successful. Christopher is sleeping through the night and getting himself back to sleep if he wakes.

Looking to the future, if he begins waking again, Mother plans to begin with small steps again – checking on him in person until she feels comfortable just calling to him.

Cry It Out Approach

The second family we will look at includes Karin, age ten months, and her parents. Karin's problem with early rising is a new one that her parents would like to solve quickly. They have chosen to stop responding to her during the early waking and let her cry-it-out.

Gather Data   Karin's parents look at both past and present events.

Sleep history: Karin began sleeping 8 hours a night at six months and 10 hours by the time she was eight months old.

Current sleep patterns: At nine months, she began waking once at 5:00 a.m. Her parents guess that this is in response to two things: the shift from British Summer Time to GMT and her learning to stand on her own.

Expectations: For her age she should have 10 hours of uninterrupted sleep: from 9:00 p.m. until 7:00 a.m.

Define the Problem

Karin's parents see one major concern:

- Difficulty getting through the early morning arousal.

Long-term goals: Karin will sleep all night and learn to get back to sleep on her own.

Look at Alternatives

Karin's parents review both small scale approaches and major ones.

Small-scale approaches: *Stabilize daytime routine* – be sure to keep regular nap schedules and minimize daytime and evening stimulation. *Teach her to get down from standing position* – during the day, show her that she will not get hurt if she 'plops' down on a soft landing.

Major-scale approaches: Karin's parents think that either crying it out or teaching her in small steps might work.

Decide on a Plan

Both Karin's parents feel confident that she can return to her old sleep patterns if they do not encourage her waking by reinforcing it. Since it does not seem to be an ingrained habit, they will attempt to make changes all at once by letting her cry.

Put the Plan into Action

Karin's parents give thought to how their decision could best be implemented.

Set the scene: Check her cot for safety and softness; make sure she is warm and comfortable when they put her down. Hang blankets over the window to decrease morning light and towels around the door to absorb some noise for the sake of the rest of the family.

Plan in action: Dad puts her to bed with the regular routine of singing and 'reading' a story. Since he puts her to bed, it is decided ahead of time he will check on her when she wakes in the early morning to be sure she is not ill or caught somehow.

After putting her to bed, he says 'goodnight', and leaves. She cries for 30 minutes, quiets down, and then begins crying again. He chooses not to go to her. She cries for another 15 minutes and goes to sleep.

The next morning she wakes again at 5:00 a.m. He checks on her and uses the same tactic. She cries for 30 minutes and goes to sleep. The next morning she surprises them by crying hard for 45 minutes – they had expected her to cry for a shorter time. They decide to continue their plan until the pattern breaks. To their surprise, the next morning she does not wake until 7:00 a.m. The new pattern has continued.

Evaluate the Situation   Karin's parents feel they have met their goal. Karin is no longer waking at 5:00 a.m., or if she is, she has learned to go back to sleep.

Since Karin is still young, they expect her schedule to change periodically. However, they wish to remain firm in avoiding early rising and plan to respond similarly if need be.

Family Bed Approach

Shelley (age four) and her parents are the next family we will look at. Shelley's parents have weighed her current emotional needs and their own immediate need for sleep. In an effort to meet all their needs, they will create a new shared-sleeping environment

Gather Data   Shelley's parents collect both current and past data.

Sleep history: Shelley has never been an easy sleeper. As an infant she needed to be nursed to sleep at bedtime and during the night. As a toddler she was easily stimulated and needed a long ritual to ease her into sleep. If she woke during the night, it usually only took a short visit from her mother or father before she returned to sleep.

Current sleep patterns: She has begun expressing many fears during the day. When she wakes at night it is no longer a quick process to get her back to sleep. She comes to her parents' bed. They return her to her own, settle her down, only to be greeted by her again. This happens several times each night and has recently developed into an angry power struggle. Her parents give in and allow her to stay with them. Not only do they feel they have lost the battle, but they have difficulty sleeping with a squirming child. To get to sleep, dad just moves to Shelley's bed.

Expectations: Shelley's parents understand that fears are common at this age. They don't mind comforting her, but would like their own sleep to be less disturbed.

Define the Problem

Shelley's parents find two areas of concern:

- Frequent waking.
- Difficulty sleeping alone.

Long-term goal: Everyone in the family will sleep soundly.

Short-term goals: Offer Shelley the comfort she needs until her fears subside; encourage her not to wake others.

Look at Alternatives

Both small scale approaches and major changes are considered.

Small-scale approaches: *Stabilize daytime routine* – keep routines simple and predictable. Keep bedtime early to prevent Shelley from becoming overtired. *Fears* – teach Shelley how to handle nightmares when they occur. Uncover and try to eliminate the source of her fears.

Major-scale approaches: Shelley's parents consider the following approaches: Family Bed, Cry It Out, and Live With It.

Decide on a Plan

Shelley's parents feel that letting her cry it out would add unnecessary trauma – besides, she brings her crying to them. Living with it is out – they've already found that unworkable. For now, their need for sleep requires immediate action. A modified Family Bed plan is their choice.

Put the Plan into Action Putting the plan into action is relatively easy for Shelley's parents.

Set the scene: Since having Shelley in their own bed disturbs everyone, they set up a temporary sleeping area in their room for her.

Plan in action: Shelley begins the night in her own room with the understanding that she can move to her new spot if she needs to. The first three nights, Shelley comes to their room upset. After some comforting, she settles into her new spot for the rest of the night. The fourth night, they hear her wake, but she quietly settles into her new spot. This continues and the family's sleep is markedly improved.

Evaluate the Situation Shelley's parents are happy with the results of their plan: Shelley's need for comfort is being met and their own sleep is much less disturbed.

After a few months her fears subside greatly. She begins sleeping in her own room all night on occasion. They discuss the possibility of offering a reward for those nights, but decide against it. Instead, they begin, in a matter-of-fact way, to say that someday she probably will want to stay in her own room all night. They plant the idea in her mind and let it take its own course. They feel confident that it will. Now that they are getting enough sleep and Shelley is less frightened, they feel no sense of urgency.

Future plan: They will keep Shelley's special spot until she suggests they dismantle it. Should she return to frequent usage, they will let it go unnoticed so that it will not be reinforced either positively or negatively by them.

Living With It Approach

The fourth family we will look at consists of Carolyn (age three), Amanda (two months), and their parents. Carolyn has begun waking at night screaming. Her parents hope that these disturbances are related to developmental changes and will pass if they live with it.

Gather Data   Carolyn's parents look at past and present patterns.

Sleep history: Carolyn has had predictable, easy-to-handle sleep patterns most of her life.

Current sleep patterns: Carolyn has begun waking at night, screaming and crying. Although she calls out, she doesn't seem to want her parents. Two things in her life have changed: she has a new baby sister and she has just given up her afternoon nap.

Expectations: Her parents would like her to return to sleeping throughout the night without waking. She may be a bit earlier than most children in giving up her nap, but it is within the norm.

Define the   Carolyn's parents find three areas of concern:
Problem
• Carolyn's distress and safety when she wakes.
• Her waking disrupts other family members' sleep.

After charting her sleeping/waking patterns for a week, Carolyn's parents see a telltale pattern. She 'wakes' near the end of her deep sleep segment – about 11:00 p.m. They define the problem as sleep terrors.

Long-term goal: Carolyn will outgrow the difficulty.

Short-term goal: Parents will keep her safe during the incidents.

Look at   Both small-scale approaches and major changes are looked
Alternatives   at.

Small-scale approaches: Carolyn's parents have learned that well-rested children have smoother sleep cycles. *Stabilize daytime routine* – continue to offer quiet time in the afternoons. Decrease stimulation during the day and at bedtime. Make bedtime early. *Check sleep environment* – make an effort to soundproof Carolyn's bedroom to decrease the chance of waking her baby sister. Move the bedside table (with sharp corners) away from her bed for safety.

Major-scale approaches: Her parents consider just living with it until Carolyn grows out of sleep terrors.

Decide on a Plan

They decide to live with it. Since Mother is frequently awake nursing the baby, Father will respond to Carolyn. He will go to her quickly, offer her a dummy and blanket. If she cannot accept his comfort, he will step back and allow her to work through it on her own. If she gets out of bed, he will gently encourage her to stay in her room, and lead her back to bed, if possible. They decide they will not discuss the incident with her in the morning.

Put the Plan into Action

Carolyn's parents begin their plan right away.

Set the scene: They 'soundproof' Carolyn's room with a rug on the floor and a blanket tacked up on the door. They move any furniture with sharp edges away from her bed.

Plan in action: Carolyn has a sleep terror about three times a week. Once she climbed out of bed, then dropped to the floor to go back to sleep! She screamed and flailed for half an hour only one night during the first month. Most often, she accepted her dummy and settled down quickly.

Evaluate the Situation

Although Carolyn's parents are still very tired, they feel confident in their approach now that they have learned more about sleep terrors. They had been worried that the waking was due to emotional distress over the new baby. They no longer take her waking during the night personally, nor are they angry at her. Because they have made a plan and are following through with it they don't feel so powerless anymore.

One Problem, Four Solutions

Now let's look at how one family might carry out each of the four major approaches. In the six steps of problem

solving, the information gathering step and problem definition will be the same for each approach. It is in the goal
setting and implementation steps that differences will be
obvious.

Gather Data   Again, we will look at the background of the problem, and
then at what the parents would like to change. Scott is a year
and a half old. He typically wakes three to four times a
night. His parents have morning responsibilities and need
more uninterrupted sleep.

History: Scott has never been a sound sleeper. Repeated
respiratory infections have kept him up at night. His parents
rocked him in order to keep him in an upright position for
easier breathing. Consequently, he has never 'slept through
the night'.

Current sleep patterns: Scott is out of critical
respiratory danger. He still wakes once or twice a night.
Rocking doesn't work anymore because he squirms and
wants to play.

Expectations for his age: 10 to 12 hours a night with
occasional waking.

Define the   Let's assess the problem areas.
Problem
• Concern over stability of Scott's health.
• Frequent waking and difficulty falling back to sleep after
waking.
• Parents' sleep is interrupted.
• Scott seems to need parents' presence, but is only stimu-
lated by their attempts to get him back to sleep.

SOLUTION 1:   Let's look at how Scott's parents might decide on and use
Family Bed   the Family Bed.

Review goals: *Long-term goal* – Scott will eventually
sleep all night in his own bed when he is ready. *Short-term
goal* – parents will get more sleep.

Look at alternatives: Scott's parents begin to look at
small-scale alternatives and changes. *Medical consultation*

– the doctor agrees Scott should be sleeping better. He says that Scott's health will benefit from predictable, uninterrupted sleep. If Scott is healthy, allowing him to cry for reasonable periods of time will not be harmful. *Stabilize daytime routine* – keep schedule simple and predictable. Keep bedtime early enough to prevent Scott from becoming overly tired.

Decide on a plan: The doctor's opinion helps motivate Scott's parents to find a way for Scott to get more sleep. They do not want to push him to go back to sleep by himself if he isn't ready. They know themselves that they would have a hard time letting him cry it out. They decide to try a modified Family Bed plan. They will offer reassurance without stimulation.

Set the scene: Scott's parents look at what they need to do to prepare for the plan and then to put it into action. They set up a carry-cot next to their bed. Next, they tell Scott about the carry-cot and let him pretend to sleep there during the day.

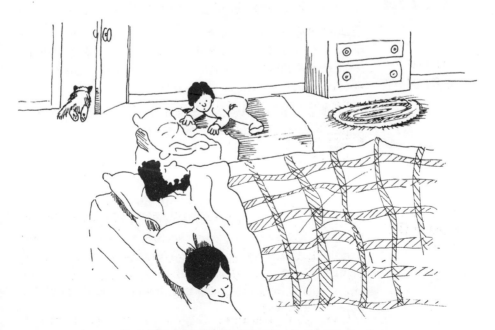

A modified Family Bed plan works for this family.

Plan in action: The first night, Scott wakes up in his own bed. His father brings him to the cot. He is somewhat excited by the new arrangement, but responds to Mother talking quietly to him and rubbing his back – which she can do from her own bed. He falls asleep after 30 minutes. He wakes once more, but responds to Mother's request to go back to sleep.

The second night, he wakes once, is put in the carry-cot and goes back to sleep. He wakes again, but responds quickly to his Mother's request to go back to sleep.

The third night he does not wake at all. The fourth night he goes back to sleep immediately when he is put into the carry-cot.

Evaluate the situation: Scott's parents have reached their short-term goal. All parties are getting more sleep – interrupted, but not for long. They caution themselves that, in order to reach their long-term goal, they must continue to be as 'boring' as possible during the night.

SOLUTION 2:
Cry it Out

We will now look at how Scott's parents might solve the sleep problem using the Cry It Out approach.

Review goals: *Long-term goal* – Scott will sleep all night or be able to get himself back to sleep after waking. *Short-term goal* – Scott will learn new sleep associations that do not involve his parents.

Look at alternatives: Scott's parents look at some small scale alternatives and changes. *Medical consultation* – as before, the doctor agrees Scott should be sleeping better. We know that Scott's health will improve with predictable, uninterrupted sleep. If Scott is not sick, allowing him to cry for reasonable periods of time will not hurt him. *Stabilize daytime routine* – again, keep schedule routine as simple as possible. Keep bedtime early so that Scott won't become overtired. *Attachment to love objects* – Scott has a favourite blanket. He begins to learn to associate it with comfort and sleep when Mother includes it in his bedtime ritual and in other quiet times.

Decide on a plan: The doctor's assurance encourages

Scott's parents to find a fast solution. They agree that everyone can handle some short-term pain if the result is more sleep – so they decide to try the Cry It Out approach.

Set the scene: Scott's parents look at the physical setting; they check Scott's cot for safety and stability. Since Scott usually cries for Mother first, they agree that she will deal with him. The parents agree to support each other during his crying.

As for timing, they agree to start the plan on a weekend, so the lost sleep is less important for all concerned, and so both parents are available to Scott during the day for positive experiences. They feel this approach will reinforce Scott positively for his hard work and alleviate some of their own discomfort.

Lastly, they talk to Scott about the plan and what will happen.

Plan in action: They decide to give the plan one week – although they hope it will not take that long to work. The first night, Mother uses the newly established routine to put Scott to bed. She makes sure Scott's favourite blanket is present. She says 'Night-night, now' and leaves the room. Scott falls asleep.

He wakes once at 4:00 a.m. Mother checks on him to make sure he isn't ill or hasn't hurt himself. She says 'Night-night, now,' lays him back down and leaves the room. Scott cries for 20 minutes, quiets down, and then begins crying again. Mother chooses not to go to Scott again; she knows he isn't ill or hurt, and wants him to learn to go back to sleep by himself. Scott cries for another 15 minutes and then goes back to sleep.

The next night Scott wakes at 5:00 a.m. Mother checks on him and uses the same tactic. Scott cries for 25 minutes and then goes back to sleep.

The third night, he wakes up at 4:00 a.m. Mother checks on him once. Although they had expected him not to cry for long, he cries loudly for 45 minutes. But their resolve is firm; they continue the plan. To their surprise, the next night, he sleeps all the way through to 7:00 a.m. The new pattern has continued.

Evaluate the situation: Scott's parents are pleased to have reached their goal. During the night they were not sure they'd make it. Their decision to nurture Scott and themselves additionally during the day was what got them through the nights of crying.

Scott did not show adverse effects or even angry feelings during the day as they carried out the plan. They decide that if the old waking pattern begins again, they will check on him once a night and then let him draw on the resources he has learned to get back to sleep on his own.

SOLUTION 3: Teaching in Small Steps

We will now look at how Scott's parents might solve the sleep problem using the Teaching In Small Steps approach.

Review goals: *Long-term goal* – Scott will sleep all night or be able to get himself back to sleep after waking. *Short-term goal* – Scott will learn new sleep associations that do not involve his parents.

Look at alternatives: Scott's parents look at some small scale alternatives and changes. *Medical consultation* – as we know, the doctor says Scott should be sleeping better and that he will benefit from uninterrupted sleep. Allowing him to cry for reasonable amounts of time will not be harmful. *Bedtime Routine* – decide on one and use it consistently. In addition, Scott would benefit from a night light. *Stabilize daytime routine* – again, keep his schedule predictable. Make sure bedtime is set early enough to prevent Scott from becoming overly tired. *Attachment to love objects* – again, Scott has a favourite blanket. Mother will teach him to think about it in association with comfort and sleep by including it in his bedtime ritual.

Decide on a plan: The doctor's reassurance encourages Scott's parents to make some changes. Their own temperaments and their memories of what they have been through with him when he was sick led them to choose the Small Steps approach. They feel they can tolerate his crying if they are also able to check on him frequently and make sure he is all right.

Set the scene: Scott's parents look at the physical

setting; they check Scott's cot for safety and stability. Since Scott usually cries out for his mother, they agree that she will start the plan by responding to him the first night. Mother and Father will alternate nights thereafter. The parents agree to support each other during his crying.

As for timing, they agree to start the plan on a weekend, so the lost sleep is less of an issue for all concerned, and so both parents are available to Scott during the day for positive experiences. They feel this will reinforce Scott positively for his hard work and alleviate some of their own discomfort. They want him to know that cuddling can continue – just not when he is supposed to be sleeping. They talk to Scott about the plan and what will happen.

Lastly, they gather supplies for the plan: clock, paper, and pencil.

Plan in action: The first night Scott wakes at 4:00 a.m. Mother goes to him and gives him his blanket. She lays him back down with the reassuring words 'More night-night' and leaves the room. Scott hops back up and cries.

Five minutes later she comes back in and repeats the same words and actions. She uses this tactic at increasing intervals of time: 7 minutes, 10 minutes, and 15 minutes. Fifteen minutes was the planned maximum amount of time before checking on him again, but Scott continues to cry. After three 15-minute sessions, he quiets down to a whimper. Mother does not go into his room again, and he falls asleep.

The next night he wakes three times. Father begins checking at the same time intervals with a maximum of 20 minutes: check, wait 5 minutes, check, wait 7 minutes, check, wait 10 minutes, check, wait 15 minutes, check, wait 20 minutes. The first waking takes up to two 20-minute waiting sessions. The second waking (this time beginning at a 7-minute wait) also takes up to two 20-minute sessions. At the third waking, he falls asleep after the 10- minute check.

The third night he wakes once. Beginning with a 10-minute wait, Mother checks up to one 25-minute wait. He falls asleep after that.

The fourth night he wakes once. Father checks on him up to the 10-minute wait. Scott surprises his parents by quieting down soon after. Father resists checking on him for half an hour. When he does, and finds him asleep; he is optimistic about the next night.

When he wakes on the fifth night, his parents, exhausted, call to him 'Night-night' from their own room. Scott settles down after a few minutes. This continues for the next few nights, until he stops waking completely.

Evaluate the situation: Scott and his parents have reached their goal: he is now sleeping through the night with only occasional waking. Although their own sleep was disrupted because of the crying, tension, and checking, Scott's parents feel that reaching their goal was worth it. If he begins waking again, they plan to simply call 'Night-night' to him and see if that is sufficient.

SOLUTION 4: Living With It

Scott's parents decide to look at how they might live with the problem.

Review goals: *Long-term goal* – Scott will eventually sleep all night in his own bed when he is ready. *Short-term goal* – work gradually toward developing independent sleep associations. Continue to assess Scott's readiness to make a change. Find ways to make the current situation tolerable for all family members.

Look at alternatives: Scott's parents look at some small scale alternatives and changes. *Medical consultation* – again, we know the doctor agrees Scott should be sleeping better and that he will benefit from smoother sleep. *Bedtime Routine* – establish one and use it routinely. *Check environment* – eliminate possible waking factors. In addition, a night light would probably help. *Stabilize daytime routine* – again, keeping Scott's schedule simple and predictable will help. Keep bedtime early. *Attachment to love objects* – Mother begins to teach Scott to associate his favourite blanket with sleep by including it in his bedtime ritual and in special, quiet times.

Decide on a plan: Scott's parents are relieved to learn that his health is stable. They decide that, due to his medical history, he hasn't had enough of a chance to learn to sleep through the night on his own. They feel that given time, he will grow out of his night time waking. In the meantime, they decide to Live With It.

Set the scene: Scott's parents check his room to make sure his bed and the temperature are comfortable, the night light is nearby, and his special blanket is available to him. They decide to divide up the night-time duty; Mother will handle Scott during the week and Father will handle him during the weekends.

In order to support themselves, Mother will arrange time away for herself two mornings a week, and once a weekend. Father will arrange time for himself one morning a weekend and time for themselves as a couple one weekend evening a month.

They decide to respond to Scott by putting him to bed each night in his own room with the supportive assumption that he will sleep all night.

Plan in action: Scott's parents consistently use their new bedtime routine with faith that it will decrease his reliance on them at night. They do the least that is necessary to return him back to sleep during the night. They reward him for the nights that he sleeps all the way through. They reward themselves with self-nurturing during the day and encourage each other to take naps.

Evaluate the situation: Scott continues to wake once or twice a night for several weeks. Occasionally, he doesn't wake at all.

Scott's parents decide that their coping measures are adequate and that giving Scott time to learn to sleep well is important. They decide to continue with their current plan for three months and then to re-evaluate his progress and their goals.

Summary   In each scenario Scott's parents took the same initial situation, defined the problem as they saw it, and chose a plan accordingly. They reached their goals in different ways. None of the solutions were purely 'textbook', but instead were personalized to fit their own values and the child's needs and temperament. In reality, that is often how sleep problems are successfully addressed. The solution may *sound* complicated, but it needn't be. You set your goal, then use information and instinct to reach it.

One important factor is the parents themselves. We have already discussed parents' readiness and family values. Next, we will discuss feelings that can affect decision-making and follow-through.

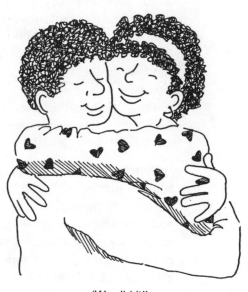

'We did it!'

Additional Reading   *Dr Spock on Parenting* by Benjamin Spock, M.D. Michael Joseph, London, 1989.

The Family Bed: An Age-old Concept in Childrearing by Tine Thevenin. Avery Publishing Group, Wayne, NJ, 1987. UK distributor: Worldwide Media Service, Partridge Green, W. Sussex RH13 8LD.

The First Three Years of Life by Burton L. White, M.D. W. H. Allen, London, 1978.

Healthy Sleep Habits, Happy Child by Marc Weissbluth, M.D. Fawcett Columbine, New York, 1987. UK distributor: Tiptree Book Services, Tiptree, Colchester CO5 0SR.

Nighttime Parenting: How to Get Your Baby and Child to Sleep by William Sears, M.D. New American Library, New York, 1987. UK distributor: Penguin Books, Harmondsworth, UB7 0DA.

To Listen to a Child by T. Berry Brazelton, M.D. Addison-Wesley, Reading, MA, 1984. UK distributor: Southport Book Distributors, Southport PR9 9YF.

Your Baby and Child: From Birth to Age Five by Penelope Leach. Michael Joseph, London, 1977.

The Womanly Art of Breastfeeding by La Leche League International. New American Library, New York, 1987. UK distributor: Penguin Books, Harmondsworth, UB7 0DA.

Chapter 7 THE PARENT'S SIDE

Parenting is not easy! Your own difficult, confusing emotions can stand in the way of constructive action. The aim of this chapter is to help you wrestle with and sort out those feelings. Guilt is often the *most* troublesome.

Guilt

I feel so many things – resentful, angry, exhausted, but most of all, guilty. Guilty when I try to make changes, and guilty when I can't follow through.

Guilt comes in many forms: guilt over letting your child cry, guilt over letting him into your bed, or guilt over not being in control. It is marked by self-doubt and self-blame. It feels like a 'no win' situation. It breeds anger – and it keeps you stuck.

Feelings of guilt arise when you sense you are not doing what you think you 'should' be doing. Look at your own set of 'shoulds'. Where did they come from? With what you *now* know about sleep, are they still valid? Go through Exercise 7.1 to sort out your own 'shoulds' and guilt-makers.

Three Kinds of Guilt

There are three kinds of guilt: self-defeating, constructive, and motivating.

Self-defeating guilt keeps you stuck, keeps you from venturing out. You become mired in your own feelings until you lose track of the real issue.

I worried so long about how miserable we both were when he was crying that I forgot how miserable we all were without sleep. The problem just continued.

Most often, guilt is a 'smoke screen' for other emotions. Sorting them out defuses the guilt and gets you back on track.

113

EXERCISE 7.1: Guilty or not Guilty?

Part one: Complete these thoughts.

1. *I feel guilty when . . .*

2. *I feel guilty because I should/shouldn't . . .*

Part two: Re-examine your expectations.

Go back to question number two. Ask yourself, 'Who says so?' Do you really agree? If so, is there a way to meet that expectation in a way that won't hinder sleep progress? If not, toss out that expectation and replace it with a new one that works better.

Sample answers:

Part one: 1. 'I feel guilty when I let him cry.' 2. 'I feel guilty because a mother *should* "be there" for her children, to help them feel better.'

Part two: 'I want him to feel safe and secure. I guess I could make extra sure during the day that he feels secure. Maybe instead of letting him cry completely alone, I could go to him and reassure him periodically.'

Constructive guilt serves a positive purpose if it *keeps* you from doing something you truly feel is wrong. You feel guilt *before* you act, but you don't *dwell* on it. To understand the difference, consider this scenario: you feel self-defeating guilt after you have eaten an entire box of biscuits – it does you no good and adds to your misery. Constructive guilt (you know what you need to do, even though you may not *want* to) steers you, instead, to the celery.

I feel so guilty bringing her into my bed that it's just not worth it. Now I patiently take her back to her own bed all the while muttering that I'll respect myself in the morning!

Motivating guilt is 'feeling guilty about feeling guilty'. For many people guilt is so ingrained it is hard to get rid of. Use your ability to feel guilty for your own purposes – teach yourself to feel guilty *about* feeling guilty.

I feel guilty when he cries – oops – I mean, I'll feel guilty if I don't teach him to sleep better, even if that means he protests.

Short Term Pain <u>vs</u> Long Term Gain

To get from inaction to action, weigh the pros and cons. See if all the reasons for doing something outweigh the guilt you feel in the meantime.

The more confident you are in your goal, the easier it is to decrease the guilt. Arm yourself with information. If you are not confident, re-evaluate your goal or choice of action. If it bothers you so much that you are wracked with guilt, don't do it – find another way.

If you are confident about your goal and plan but hearing your child cry is your guilt-producer, remember that crying is a child's honest expression of frustration and anger. People get angry when they don't get what they want. *Your child has the right to express his anger without your feeling guilty.*

Summary of Guilt

Guilt is a powerful emotion and the most common one expressed by parents working on sleep habits. Guilt can lead to anger and resentment because feeling guilty implies that you are doing something wrong. Your child, partner, or someone else can become the target for feelings that are boiling beneath the surface. Then guilt begets more guilt because you think you 'shouldn't' feel or act that way.

Kind, thoughtful people are usually those most plagued by guilt because they don't like to upset others – and children who don't want to sleep *are* upset. Trust your maturity. Think of other examples when you do what is best

---

EXERCISE 7.2: Getting Rid of Self-Defeating Guilt

You can change guilt by beginning to think of your feelings in different ways. Get past the generalized guilt and recognize the specific feelings behind it. Go back to Exercise 7.1 and replace the word guilt with another emotion. Use as many as you can.

These revised feelings are usually easier to deal with than guilt. List some ways you might handle the revised feelings – or ways you have handled the same feelings in other circumstances.

Example:

Old feeling: *I feel **guilty** when he cries.*

Revised feeling: *I feel **sad** (or torn apart, helpless, nervous, frustrated) when he cries.*

Possible actions: *When I feel sad **I could** cry and ask my partner to hold me. When I feel nervous **I could** take a walk or scrub the floor.*

Your concern:

Old feeling: *I feel guilt when:*

Revised feeling: *I feel*

Possible actions: *When I feel*

   I could:

   or:

   or:

without feeling guilty (e.g. you don't let him watch the scary movie even though he pleads or screams).

To help keep perspective, remember your long term goal. For more encouragement, remember that Dr Weissbluth strongly feels that it is as important for parents to teach good sleep habits as it is to teach good nutrition and hygiene habits.

Caring for Yourself

When a child is not sleeping, parents who are usually calm and rational find their minds can be muddled from lack of sleep. Raw emotions often rise to the surface.

He keeps me awake all night, then greets me with a smile and wants a hug in the morning. I grit my teeth and try to make it through the day until naptime. I try to figure out what to do . . . but I just end up crying. I'm so tired!

You cannot take care of your children until you take care of yourself. This is not a cliché, or something to put off until the kids are older. Getting yourself to the frame of mind (and body) where you can 'take charge' needs to be your number one priority.

Nurturing yourself is cumulative; instead of dreaming of a week on the beach in Hawaii, do little things for yourself each day. If you have chosen to live with a sleep problem, there are more tips in the Living With It section of this book. If you are still struggling with the problem and can't seem to sort it through, take steps to build up your emotional and physical stamina before you proceed. If you are ready to begin a plan, build some self nurturing into the plan.

Nurturing yourself *will* help you succeed. Here are some ideas to consider.

- Give yourself permission to sleep during the day. No one is watching.
- Check your nutrition. Are you eating right? If not, you will tire more easily.
- Get regular exercise and fresh air. You need this as much as your child.
- Adjust your bedtime, if needed. Turn off your phone.
- Find some time for you alone. Not easy to do? Practice

EXERCISE 7.3: Defuse Guilt

Defuse guilt by checking it against your values and goals. Go back to Exercise 7.1. Weigh the 'because' of part two against your long-term goal (in step 2 of Exercise 5.2 in Chapter 5).

Example 1:

Guilt: *I feel guilty because a good mother should comfort her child when she is distraught.*

Goal: *To teach positive sleep habits.*

Weigh the two: *A good mother also teaches good sleep habits. Perhaps my child will be distraught for a shorter time if we work towards that goal.*

Example 2:

Guilt: *I feel guilty letting her sleep with us because I can just hear my mother say, 'You'll never get her out of your bed!'*

Goal: *I want to get some sleep!*

Weigh the two: *I need sleep and I feel good when she sleeps near me. My child is sleeping here, not my mother.*

Your concern:

Guilt:

Goal:

Weigh the two:

taking time 'alone' with your child: put her in a stroller and walk fast; turn on a children's tape when you drive so they are less likely to talk to you.

- Pamper yourself at least as much as you pamper your child – it's a good rule of thumb.
- Seriously consider all offers of help – from the sales assistant at the supermarket to your mother-in-law.

- Change your standards – for your house, yourself, and your partner.
- Practise saying aloud good things about yourself – or ask a friend to say them to you.
- Re-evaluate your priorities – put yourselves individually, and as a couple, higher on the list.

Where to Go When Nothing Works

If you are still troubled by sleep problems, look for outside professional help. Start with your child's doctor. He or she can refer you to a specialist, if needed. If there is a hospital nearby, they can help you find an appropriate specialty – from neurology to behavioural sciences. Some universities have sleep study programmes and may offer help.

Your local library is a good resource. Ask for the research centre's directory to see if there is a centre nearby – or one close enough to consult by phone or mail.

Your doctor may decide to refer your child to a psychologist. Psychologists deal more with emotional problems and help with behavioural change. Ask for one who has specialized in the area of sleep.

When you are embroiled in the problem, angry because the situation is out of control, and exhausted from lack of sleep, it is hard to think through and carry out a plan. Sometimes just talking to a neutral person can help you gain the objectivity you need. Please don't suffer alone.

Conclusion

A good night's rest: it is important to all of us, child and adult alike. Sleeping well doesn't come naturally or spontaneously to everyone. It is a skill that can be learned and can be taught.

Stop for a moment and realize how far you have already come. Even though *you* are exhausted, you have finished reading this book. You have gained a basic understanding of children's sleep. You have begun to apply this information to your specific situation – you have defined the problem, sorted out the underlying issues, and assessed your values and goals. You are ready to make your decision, and you are committed to making it work.

It may take some time and it may take some hard work for all of you, but the results will be worth it.

Good night!

Additional Readings

Healthy Sleep Habits, Happy Child, by Marc Weissbluth, MD. Fawcett Columbine, New York, 1987. UK distributor: Tiptree Book Services, Tiptree, Colchester CO5 0SR.

The Parent/Child Sleep Guide. Sleep Products Safety Council/Better Sleep Council, P.O. Box 13, Washington, DC 20044.

End Notes

Chapter 1   [1] White, Burton, M.D. *The First Three Years of Life*. W. H. Allen, London, 1978.
[2] Weissbluth, Marc, M.D. *Healthy Sleep Habits, Happy Child*. Fawcett Columbine, New York: 1987.

Chapter 2   [1] Ferber, Richard, M.D. *Solve Your Child's Sleep Problems*. Dorling Kindersley, London, 1986.
[2] ibid.
[3] Weissbluth, Marc, M.D. *Healthy Sleep Habits, Happy Child*. Fawcett Columbine, New York: 1987.

Chapter 3   [1] Brazelton, T. Berry, M.D. *To Listen to a Child*. Addison-Wesley, Reading, MA: 1984.
[2] Ferber, Richard, M.D. *Solve Your Child's Sleep Problems*. Dorling Kindersley, London, 1986.

Chapter 4   [1] Thevenin, Tine. *The Family Bed: An Age-old Concept in Childrearing*. Avery Publishing Group, Wayne, NJ: 1987.

Bibliography

Brazelton, T. Berry, M.D. *To Listen to a Child*. Reading, MA: Addison-Wesley, 1984. UK distributor: Southport Book Distributors, Southport PR9 9YF.

Cuddigan, Maureen and Mary Beth Hanson. *Growing Pains: Helping Children Deal with Everyday Problems through Reading*. Chicago: American Library Assoc., 1988. UK distributor: International Book Distributors, Hemel Hempstead HP2 4RG.

Ferber, Richard, M.D. *Solve Your Child's Sleep Problems*. London: Dorling Kindersley, 1986.

Garfield, Patricia, Ph.D. *Your Child's Dreams*. New York: Ballantine, 1984. UK distributor: Tiptree Book Services, Tiptree, Colchester CO5 0SR.

La Leche League International. *The Womanly Art of Breastfeeding*. New York: New American Library, 1987. UK distributor: Penguin Books, Harmondsworth UB7 0DA.

Leach, Penelope. *Your Baby and Child: From Birth to Age Five*. London: Michael Joseph, 1977.

Sears, William, M.D. *Nighttime Parenting: How to Get Your Baby and Child to Sleep*. New York: New American Library, 1987. UK distributor: Penguin Books, Harmondsworth UB7 0DA.

Sleep Products Safety Council. *The Parent/Child Sleep Guide*. Washington, DC: Sleep Products Safety Council/ Better Sleep Council, P.O. Box 13, Washington, DC 20044.

Spock, Benjamin, M.D. *Dr Spock on Parenting*. London: Michael Joseph, 1989.

Thevenin, Tine. *The Family Bed: An Age-old Concept in Childrearing*. Wayne, NJ: Avery Publishing Group, 1987. UK distributor: Worldwide Media Service, Partridge Green, W. Sussex RH13 8LD.

Weissbluth, Marc, M.D. *Healthy Sleep Habits, Happy Child*. New York: Fawcett Columbine, 1987. UK distributor: Tiptree Book Services, Tiptree, Colchester CO5 0SR.

White, Burton L., M.D. *The First Three Years of Life*. London: W. H. Allen, 1978.

Wiseman, Anne Sayre. *Nightmare Help – For Children, From Children*. Berkeley, CA: Ten Speed Press, 1989. UK distributor: Airlift Book Company, 26–28 Eden Grove, London N7 8EF.

Family Bed Approach

Summary from *The Sleep Book For Tired Parents*

Parents welcome the child or children into the parental bed for shared sleep. Children spend as much or as little time as they need in the 'family bed'.

Philosophy

Parents want to be available for children during the night as during the day. They can meet the needs of children without leaving their own bed, so sleep is minimally disturbed. The infant and mother develop a mutual sleep cycle; and the infant can nurse as desired. An older child need not face separation at sleep time. Fears are calmed by the parents' presence. Father is nearby.

Arrangements are highly individualized. They range from all members sleeping together all the time, to children welcome only in special circumstances.

Procedure

Decide on a sleeping arrangement that allows everyone to sleep most comfortably.

- Who will sleep where?
- What are the special circumstances or conditions?
- Does the child also have his own room and bed? How and when will it be used?

Make the necessary arrangements – an infant can simply be brought to your bed; older or multiple children may take more planning. Options might be:

- Buy or build a bigger bed.
- Set up cots or sleeping bags nearby.

Establish ground rules:

- How will bedtime be handled?
- When are children allowed in parental bed? (always, when frightened, etc.)
- How will parents' need for privacy be met?
- What is the time frame? (until infancy passes, until child decides, etc.)

Two Families Proceed

Infant Carl sleeps between his parents. His room will be used primarily for play and keeping his things until he is older and chooses to move to his own bed. Carl's parents decide to respond to criticism with a smile and the comment, 'This is what works for us – Carl's needs are being met and we're all getting the sleep we need.'

Elizabeth is welcome in her parents' bed when she feels she needs them – when she is frightened or ill. She always begins the night in her own room, and the expectation is that she stay there most of the time. As she grows older she will come less often to her parents' room.

Cry It Out Approach

Summary from *The Sleep Book For Tired Parents*

Parents do not respond to the child while he learns to put himself to, or back to, sleep. This usually involves crying for as long as necessary each time – most often taking about three days or up to one week.

Philosophy

Attention from a parent reinforces behaviour. In this case, the behaviour is crying for a parent's presence and help to get back to sleep. A parent's attempt to help or check on the child will hinder his learning independent sleep habits. A child will learn to go to sleep by himself when he wakes; staying awake is not rewarded by his parents' attention or presence.

Procedure

Select a time to begin the plan when the child and parents won't need to be especially well-rested. Weekends are often good times to start.

Prepare for the discomfort crying brings. Parents need to plan ahead to cope with the setting and their own feelings. Blankets around doorways and rugs or floor covering in the child's room helps to muffle sound. Parents also plan on how to nurture and support each other during the crying.

'Explain' the plan to the child in a positive, reassuring manner. Prepare other family members or neighbours, if need be.

One Family Proceeds

At bedtime: After a simple, calming bedtime routine mum puts Andrew to bed and leaves the room. Andrew cries (if he needs to) until he falls asleep.

During the night: Two options

- Go to Andrew immediately. Check on his safety and health. Offer brief, calm words of goodnight and leave the room. He cries until he falls asleep.
- Do not go to him or respond in any way. He cries until he falls asleep. When you are certain he is asleep, check on him if you like.

While working on a problem, try to limit excess crying to sleep learning times. The child is reassured that his cries are heard and responded to as appropriate. In the morning, parents respond quickly.

Try to schedule some quiet, nurturing time for parents to interact with the child during daytime hours.

Teaching In Small Steps

Summary from *The Sleep Book For Tired Parents*

Parents decide on a goal and work backward breaking down the necessary learning into small steps, and ask the child to make changes gradually.

Philosophy

When a child is accustomed to, and attached to, her sleep habits, asking her to change them all at once is difficult. New learning done in stages allows time for adjustment to the new expectation. Parents can provide emotional support during the process.

If crying is necessary, it is broken down into a time frame that the parent feels comfortable with and the child learns from. The parent responds less frequently and is less involved, and the child is given more time to learn to settle herself. The child is not left totally alone, nor is the parent left out.

Procedure

A child can be taught to get herself to sleep when given an opportunity to settle independently of her parents. She finds and relies on her own resources to get to sleep. While she is learning, she knows parents are nearby but visits are short and they are not part of the process of going to sleep.

One Family Proceeds

Parents decide how much crying they can reasonably tolerate before checking on the child – 15 minutes is a typical maximum for the first night.

Night One:	**Night Two:**	**Night Three:**
Put child to bed.	Put child to bed.	Put child to bed.
Cries 5 minutes.	Cries 10 minutes.	Cries 15 minutes.
Parent checks.	Parent checks.	Parent checks.
Cries 10 minutes.	Cries 15 minutes.	Cries 20 minutes.
Parent checks.	Parent checks.	Parent checks.
Cries 15 minutes.	Cries 20 minutes.	Cries 25 minutes.
Parent checks.	Parent checks.	Parent checks.
Continue at 15-minute intervals until child falls asleep.	Continue at 20-minute intervals until child falls asleep.	Continue at 25-minute intervals until child falls asleep.

At Bedtime: After a calm, quiet routine, Emily is put into bed with some words of goodnight. Dad leaves the room. Emily cries for 5 minutes; dad goes to her. Without picking her up, dad offers a few words of reassurance and goodnight (taking only a minute or so) and leaves the room while she is still awake (she may not even be calmed). Dad continues waiting and checking as long as Emily cries vigorously. If the crying subsides, he need not check on her because she is starting to learn to settle herself.

During the night: For each waking they follow the same approach, beginning at 5 minutes and continuing with 15-minute intervals as needed.

Subsequent Bedtimes and wakings: Parents use the same approach – increasing the beginning and maximum interval each night. Increases continue for as many nights as is necessary until Emily is no longer crying vigorously. She may complain or whimper, but is no longer frantic. She will learn to find her blanket, suck her thumb, or 'nest' in whatever way works to get herself to sleep. During the normal night-time arousals she may cry out as she re-settles herself, but this does not require intervention.

Living With It

Summary from *The Sleep Book For Tired Parents*

Parents decide to live with the situation as it is and to develop ways to cope.

Philosophy

For personal reasons, parents feel it would not be appropriate or beneficial to make changes at this time. These reasons might include:

- A change in life circumstances, such as a move, has occurred or is expected.
- Due to the child's temperament or individual circumstances, parents feel it would be better for them to make changes than the child.
- Parents' values or temperaments indicate that there is no need for change, or that there would be no practical commitment to it.
- Parents are simply not ready yet.

Parents view *not* making a major change as a viable choice. They consciously accept it without feeling guilty or fighting it. They assess the situation and implement ways to cope. They schedule a time in the future to re-evaluate.

One Family Proceeds

Michael's parents decide that he has less need for sleep than is typical. At one year old he sleeps only six hours a night and doesn't go down for a nap. He shows no ill effects during the day. Michael's paediatrician agrees that he seems to simply need less sleep than most people.

Chart current sleep patterns. Michael is ready for bed at 1:00 a.m. and is awake again by 6:00 a.m.

Find a support system. Mum arranges for a babysitter to come in for a portion of the day to give her a break.

Develop a plan. Parents alternate staying up nights with Michael. On weekends, Dad sleeps in and Mum takes a nap. Parents plan a 'date' once a week to be by themselves and talk.

Re-evaluate plan. Parents plan to re-assess the situation at the end of each month.

Tips for Coping

- Parents alternate being 'on duty' each night of the week.
- Parents split and/or share responding to child each night.
- Divide up household chores and childcare duties between partners.
- Find help during the day to have time away from children and rejuvenate.
- Couples plan special time together away from children.
- Plan fun times with child to balance time spent in night-time caretaking.
- Stop seeking/listening to 'solutions' offered by others.

Index